GREAT MEDICAL MILESTONES

Betty Lou Kratoville

ORDER DIRECTLY FROM
H ANN ARBOR PUBLISHERS LTD.
P.O. BOX 1, BELFORD
20 Cc NORTHUMBERLAND NE70 7JX
Nov TEL. 01668 214460 FAX 01668 214484
www.annarbor.co.uk

International Standard Book Number: 1-57128-020-0

5 4 3 2 1 0 9 8 7 6
0 9 8 7 6 5 4 3 2 1

Contents

Introduction

If you were a student about to graduate from a medical school, you would be asked to take the Hippocratic Oath. It seems hard to believe that this oath was written 2500 years ago by a Greek doctor. His name was Hippocrates. This pledge sets forth high standards and ideals for anyone who plans to practice medicine.

When Hippocrates lived, medicine was in the hands of the priests. Over time he was able to stamp out many of the superstitions about illness. And he was able to move the treatment of disease away from men who knew much about religion but not about sickness.

Today many doctors agree with Hippocrates' belief that "nature heals." They also agree with his use of proper diet, fresh air, and change of climate. He stressed good habits and living conditions to his patients and students. His favorite diet for sick people was barley gruel, a cereal cooked with milk or water. His favorite medicine was honey. Today doctors use glucose – which is almost the same thing.

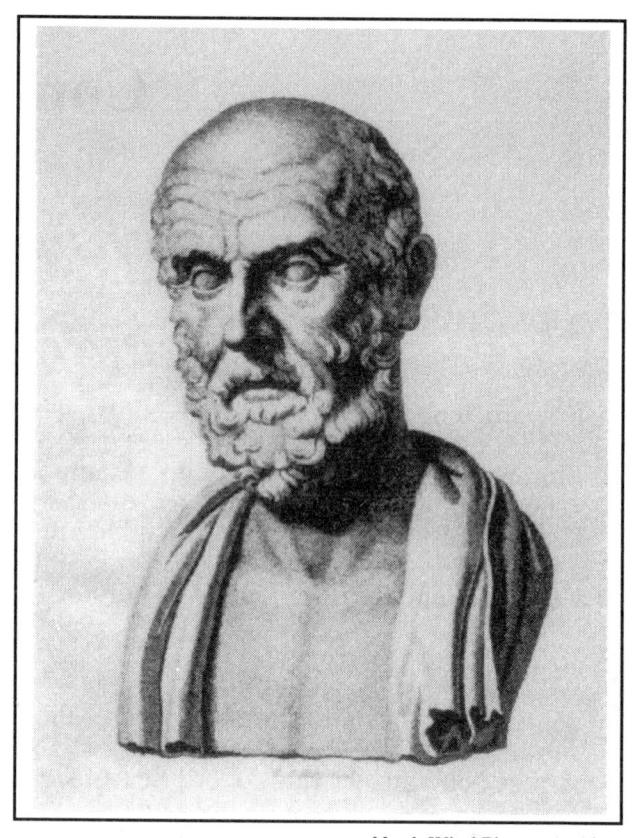

... North Wind Picture Archives

If you were a patient or a student of Hippocrates, you might meet him under a huge plane tree. This tree still stands in the town of Cos where he was born. In this open-air clinic Hippocrates taught that it is important to look at a patient as a whole person. He pointed out that the patient is more important than his disease. He believed that a good doctor helps nature to cure the patient.

His medical writings and teachings have survived to this day. No wonder he is called the "Father of Medicine."

A sense of medical history will be gained from reading about the men and women described in this book and from completing the exercises that follow each biographical sketch. However, to fully comprehend the contributions of these legendary figures, it is important that the vocabulary in each one be studied and mastered in advance. Difficult words have been underlined and should be looked up in the vocabulary section (beginning on page 67) and thoroughly discussed before any of the sketches is read for the first time. It is also recommended that vocabulary words be used in oral discussions before and after a sketch has been read so that the pronunciation and meaning become familiar.

EDWARD JENNER
Extraordinary Country Doctor

The Problem

Before the 18th Century people were terrified of smallpox. And no wonder! It was indeed one of the most dreadful diseases. It swept through countries in great <u>epidemics</u>. At such times there were barely enough well people to care for the sick. Most of the time people who got smallpox suffered and died. If they did live, they were left with ugly scars on their faces and bodies. These were called "pock-marks," and they turned goodlooking men and women into <u>repulsive</u> figures whom no one wished to be near. Sometimes smallpox also caused blindness. Many people fled from towns and cities when an epidemic struck. Often not enough people remained to bury the dead.

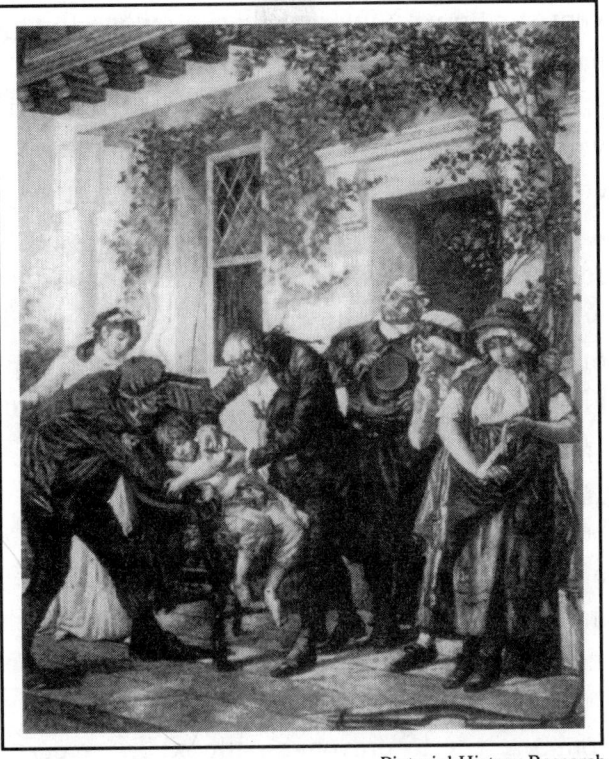

. . . Pictorial History Research

The Solution

Today we no longer need to fear smallpox. That is due to the nimble brain of a hardworking, gifted doctor. Edward Jenner was born in the English village of Berkeley in 1749. If one wanted to become a doctor in those days, one became an <u>apprentice</u> to someone who was already a doctor. This is what Edward Jenner did. He was allowed to study medicine with a surgeon, Dr. Daniel Ludlow. Dr. Ludlow must have been very impressed with the young Jenner. When Jenner was only 21, Ludlow arranged it so that he could go to London to study with the famous Dr. John Hunter. It was a rare opportunity. Hunter was a great teacher. He seemed to have a way of inspiring his students. Many of them went on to have fine careers in medicine.

Dr. Hunter put Jenner to work helping with some experiments in natural history. Among other animals they studied eels, birds, and porcupines. Because of what he had learned in the lab, Jenner was able to get a part-time job. This was necessary because his clergyman father was far from rich, and money to live on was badly needed. Jenner worked preparing <u>speci-mens</u> that had been gathered by Sir Joseph Banks on Captain Cook's first voyage in 1771. Jenner must have done a good job because he was invited to go along on Captain Cook's next long voyage.

Jenner thanked the captain and Sir Joseph but said no. He had other plans. They were quite simple. He married and returned to his home town of Berkeley. Here he practiced medicine for the rest of his life. And here he lived when he made the magnificent discovery that has benefitted all of mankind.

At this time a number of people in different countries had been trying to find a way to prevent smallpox. Now and then someone thought he had stumbled on an answer. But all efforts had failed.

The fact that a country doctor succeeded where many scientists failed happened in an odd way. One day a dairymaid said to him, "I won't ever get smallpox because I have already had cowpox." What a strange thing to say. And how did she know this?

Cowpox was a common but mild disease. People who milked cows seemed to get it. Jenner began to ask questions. He learned that many people agreed with the milkmaid. People who had been ill with cowpox did not get smallpox. He also learned that there were two kinds of cowpox. Only one of them seemed to keep dairy workers from getting smallpox. Using this knowledge, Jenner worked slowly and carefully. Finally it was time to put his <u>theories</u> to the test.

It must have taken a great deal of courage for Jenner to try out his theories on a human being. His first subject was an eight-year-old boy. Jenner <u>vaccinated</u> him with <u>pus</u> from the hand of a dairymaid who had the "right kind" of cowpox. He waited eight weeks. Then he vaccinated the boy with pus from a smallpox victim. And then the awful waiting began. Each day Jenner examined the boy. There was no sign of smallpox!

After many weeks the boy remained well. It was only then that Jenner felt that he had truly found a way to prevent smallpox. Two years later he announced his amazing discovery to the world. And, of course, the world was thrilled!

Great quantities of the <u>vaccine</u> were made at once. Perhaps too quickly because one batch of vaccine was found to be impure. A number of people grew sick from it. However, Jenner was able to locate the source of the trouble. Happily, no other problems occurred. People lined up to be vaccinated. The number of smallpox dropped year by year.

Jenner continued to lead a very simple life although many honors came his way. He had no interest in fame or money. He was offered a job in London at a huge salary. He turned it down. He said he could get along very nicely on what monies he had and did not need more. He was quite content to live and practice medicine in a small town with his wife and children and friends around him.

Later he did accept some large sums of money from the British government. He did this so that he could vaccinate free of charge all of the poor people who came to him. In good weather he used to move all of his medical equipment into the garden. There he saw poor patients. Often he vaccinated as many as 300 people in a day.

Although he hated to leave his home and village, now and then he did so for a special event. For example, Oxford University gave him high honors. He went to London and was presented to the king and queen. One story points out how international was his fame: England and France were at war. Napoleon was about to refuse to release some English prisoners of war. Just then he heard his wife Josephine mention the name of Jenner. "Ah, we can refuse nothing to that name," said Napoleon. And the prisoners were sent home to England.

Sadness entered Jenner's life. He never quite got over the fact that, as a doctor, he was unable to save the life of his eldest son who died in 1810. Five years later his wife died. Jenner was only 66 at the time but he retired from his practice and from public life. He spent the rest of his life writing books and articles. He died on January 24, 1823. leaving a safer, healthier world.

On a separate sheet of paper list all the underlined words in the story about Edward Jenner. Find them in the vocabulary section beginning on page 67. Review their meaning and pronunciation. Choose any four and write a sentence for each one.

EDWARD JENNER
In Other Words

LESSON NO. 1

Here are 12 words that appear in the story of Edward Jenner. The object of the assignment is to find words of 2, 3, 4, or more letters by using letters from each clue word IN THE SAME ORDER IN WHICH THEY APPEAR IN THE WORD.

Example: international = in (This goes in the 5 point column.)
international = it (This goes in the 10 point column.)
international = nail (This goes in the 15 point column.)

A perfect score is 360. Remember! You cannot change the order of the letters in the clue word.

Clue Word	5 Points	10 Points	15 Points
international	in	it	nail
countries			
prisoners			
vaccinated			
theories			
specimens			
medicine			
apprentice			
experiment			
opportunity			
repulsive			
disease			
Total Points			
GRAND TOTAL			

EDWARD JENNER
Activities

LESSON NO. 2

In Class

1. Write a paragraph describing the four worst things about being sick.

_____

_____

_____

_____

2. Write a paragraph describing the four best things about being sick.

_____

_____

_____

_____

At Home

1. Ask to see your medical records. Make a list of all the vaccinations and shots you have been given.

2. Find out what a "booster shot" is.

At the Library

1. Dr. Jenner became a doctor by becoming an apprentice to a surgeon. How does one become a doctor today?

2. Try to find out if there are any cases of smallpox in the world today. If so, where and why?

FLORENCE NIGHTINGALE
Lady with a Lamp

The Problem

It is hard to believe that in the 1800's military hospitals were a disgrace! It was true in the United States during the Civil War. It was true of England during the Crimean War. It simply was a fact of army life. Even men with minor wounds often died. In fact, they would not have had to suffer so much if they had been killed outright. Why was this so? Army hospitals were dirty and overcrowded. Supplies were short – few beds, no clean sheets or bandages, awful food, if any. The few doctors did not have operating tables. In those days women were banned from taking care of male patients. So there were no nurses to speak of. The wounded lay on bare floors. Often they cried out for water. But they cried out in vain. No one was there to heed their agony.

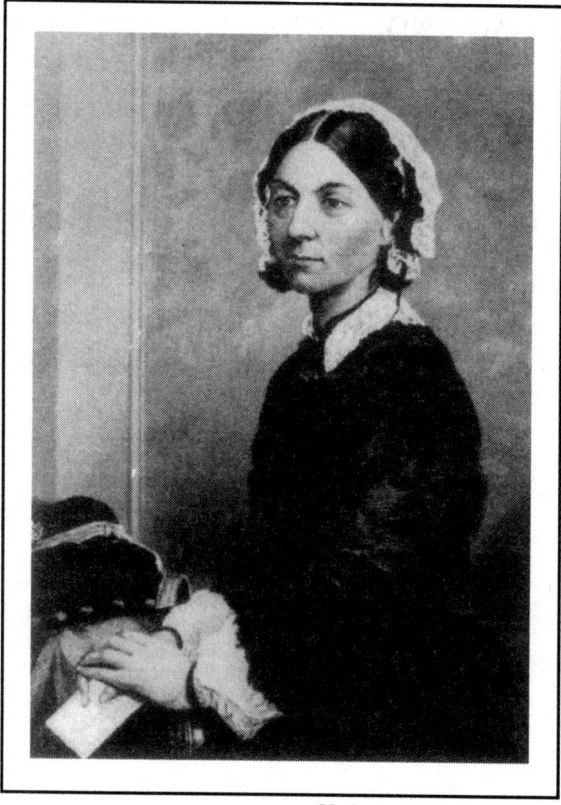

. . . Underwood Photo Archives

Civilian hospitals were no better. They were dark and dirty. Patients with all sorts of different diseases were crammed into the same ward, sometimes even the same bed. The few untrained nurses were often drunk. The system was crying out for someone who cared.

The Solution

Florence Nightingale cared. And she changed hospitals forever. It was she who began the first-rate nursing care we receive today. And she had to fight to do it. She had to fight her family and friends. They felt nursing was not proper work for a young gentlewoman. She had to fight the government. Men did not want a woman upsetting their <u>system</u> even if it was bad. But Florence Nightingale would not listen to any of them.

Florence's parents were traveling in Italy when she was born in 1820. Her family was well-to-do and had several country homes. She never went to school. Her father taught her at home. After lessons she liked to play with dolls. She often pretended they were hurt or sick. When she grew older, she cared for sick aunts and cousins. Sometimes she even looked after poor village people who were ill.

Florence and her sister were presented to the queen. There were lots of parties. She could have had a life filled with fun. But Florence wasn't interested. She had only one wish, and that was to be a nurse. After years of searching she finally heard of a hospital in Germany that took women students to train as nurses. When she got there, she found a clean hospital where patients were given fine care. It was just what she had been looking for. But it had taken her several years to convince her parents to let her go. In fact, she never really did convince them. They forbade her to tell anyone where she was going. Florence didn't care. She was on her way.

Life at the German hospital was hard. Students rose at 5:00 A.M. Simple meals lasted only 10 minutes. But Florence felt her life had meaning at long last. Later she went to Paris to study French nursing. She made dozens of notes and charts and lists. In her own way Florence was learning how a hospital should be run.

Back in London she took the post of <u>superintendent</u> at a hospital for women. The hospital was new. She had just 10 days to get ready for patients. She was everywhere at once. No detail was too small for her attention. Everyone connected with the hospital was <u>astonished</u>. They had expected changes but nothing like this. The fact was that Florence was years ahead of her time. In a very short time she became known as an expert in her field.

It was no wonder then that she was called on to help with the neglect and suffering in the <u>Crimea</u>, an area in Turkey where England was at war. She somehow collected a group of 39 nurses. Florence and her group got to the town of Scutari the same day that about 500 British soldiers were brought in. They had been wounded about 10 days before. But their wounds had not yet been given any attention. Florence could not believe her eyes. Everywhere she looked she saw pain and misery. Where were supplies, she wanted to know. It seems they had not been unloaded from ships. No one seemed to know what to do about it. Luckily, Florence was somewhat prepared. She had brought her own supplies. Conditions began to get better at once. Florence and her nurses scrubbed floors and washed the wounded. They made mattresses. They cooked good hot food. At first the doctors resented her. She and her nurses had to work carefully. They dared not offend the doctors. But at last the huge tide of wounded men worked in her favor. The doctors simply had to have her help. Then Florence and her team were free to pitch in. And pitch in they did!

The patients' clothes had not been washed in five weeks. They were covered with lice. The nurses boiled the clothes and scrubbed the men. Florence wrote an angry letter to London about supplies. Soon soap, trays, dishes, sheets, and other badly-needed items began to arrive. Now patients lived instead of died.

One other huge problem came up. Wounded men continued to pour in. There was not another inch of space for more beds. One wing of the hospital had been badly damaged by fire. It could not be used but no one seemed ready or willing to do anything about it. Finally Florence hired workers using her own money and some funds that had been <u>donated</u>.

By the spring of 1855 Florence Nightingale was worn out. What kept her going was the courage of the men. They tried not to complain. But they were homesick and afraid. Nurse Nightingale gave them hope just by moving among them. If she were too busy during the day, she made her rounds at night. A Turkish lamp lighted her way along the miles of beds. Forever after she was known as the "Lady with a Lamp."

At one point she came down with a severe fever. She lay near death for 12 days. As she grew better she was thin and frail. But she stayed at her post until the end of the war. Then and only then did she return home. Honor after honor came to her. She was the first woman to receive the British Order of Merit. But fame and honors seemed to mean little to her – except one. The British government gave her an award of $150,000. She used it to start the Nightingale Home for Nurses. The training courses given there were used as models all over the world. Even the United States government asked her advice in 1861 during the Civil War.

As she grew older, Florence would not see visitors unless they were connected with her work. She preferred to write letters and draft proposals for laws. She spent several years helping to reform public health in India. But eventually her eyes and her mind began to fail. She died in her sleep at age 90. Her splendid work was done.

On a separate sheet of paper list all the underlined words in the story about Florence Nightingale. Find them in the vocabulary section beginning on page 67. Review their meaning and pronunciation. Choose any four and write a sentence for each one.

FLORENCE NIGHTINGALE
Idioms

LESSON NO. 1

An idiom is a group of words that do not mean exactly what they say. For example, "It rained cats and dogs" means that it rained very heavily. Below are 12 underlined idioms. Write their meaning on the line under each one.

When Florence Nightingale got to the Crimea, she

1. had to put up a good front.

   _____

2. felt somewhat down in the mouth.

   _____

3. found that the doctors had a chip on their shoulders.

   _____

4. often had too many irons in the fire.

   _____

5. had to cool her heels until supplies arrived from England.

   _____

6. never had time on her hands.

   _____

7. often had to burn the candle at both ends.

   _____

8. sometimes felt she was up the creek without a paddle.

   _____

9. stayed on the job through thick and thin.

   _____

10. kept her nose to the grindstone.

    _____

11. at times must have felt that she was going around in circles.

    _____

FLORENCE NIGHTINGALE
Activities

LESSON NO. 2

In Class

1. Write a paragraph describing why you would like to become a nurse.

_____

_____

or

_____

2. Write a paragraph describing why you would NOT like to become a nurse.

_____

_____

_____

At Home

1. Ask a parent to show you how to take a temperature.

2. Check the Health Guide in your local telephone book. Choose a topic and call the number given. Ask to hear the tape on that topic. Then write 4 sentences on what you learned. (If there is no Health Guide in your area, choose three diseases, look them up in the dictionary, and copy down the definitions.)

At the Library

1. Look up what the Crimean War was all about. Who started it? Why? Who were the opponents? Who won?

2. Try to find some information about what American hospitals were like during the Civil War. Were hospitals different for prisoners?

ELIZABETH BLACKWELL
First Woman Doctor

The Problem

Think how you might feel if there were something terribly important in your life that you wanted to do. And you found that all doors were closed to you! This is what Elizabeth Blackwell faced in 1847 when she made up her mind to become a doctor.

The Solution

Medical school after medical school turned her down. They would not even give her a chance. One day a friend told her about a small medical <u>college</u> in Geneva, New York. Elizabeth sent in her <u>application</u> forms at once. Then the dean of that college made a most unusual <u>decision</u>. He decided to let the students decide whether or not to admit her. He was sure that the all-male student body would never vote to admit a female. He was wrong.

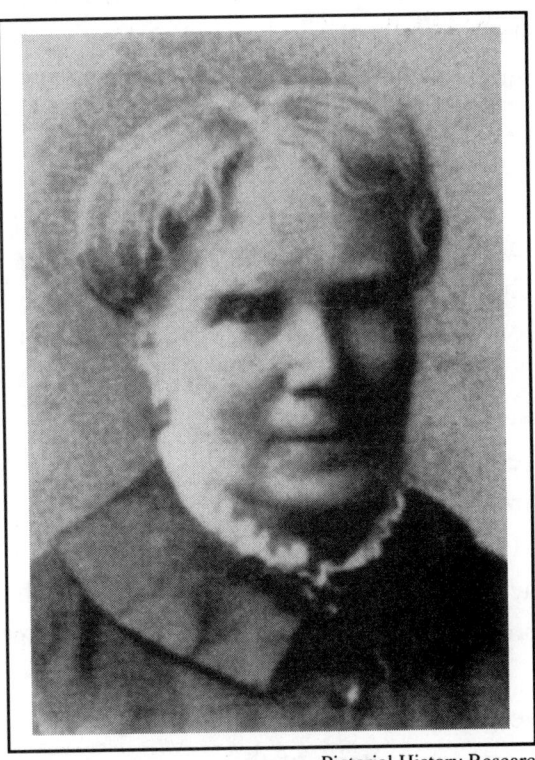

All of the students voted yes to accept Elizabeth. Their statement reads in part:

> . . . one of the <u>radical</u> <u>principles</u> of a Republican government is the <u>universal</u> education of both sexes; that to every branch of scientific education the door should be open equally to all; that the <u>application</u> of Elizabeth Blackwell to become a member of our class meets our entire <u>approbation</u>; and in extending our <u>unanimous</u> invitation we pledge ourselves that no conduct of ours shall cause her to regret her attendance at this institution.

Elizabeth's troubles, however, were not over. The town's landladies would not rent her a room. Town citizens stared rudely as she walked down the street. But at last she found someone who gave her a place to stay. She studied hard and was able to graduate in January, 1849.

Three months later Elizabeth traveled to Paris, France. Here she hoped to study surgery. Once more her hopes were dashed. Not one hospital in Paris would take a woman for <u>post-graduate</u> medical study. Again she did not give up. After a long search she found a woman's hospital that would take her as a student. She had to scrub floors, wash windows, change beds, and other <u>lowly</u> tasks. But she learned a lot about women and their medical needs.

Dr. Blackwell had more than her share of <u>obstacles</u> to overcome. A lesser person might have given up. While still in France she caught a serious eye disease from a baby for whom she was caring. This brought on blindness in her left eye. It ended any chance she might have had of becoming a surgeon. Disappointed and lonely, she came back to the United States. Here things were not a great deal better. No hospital or clinic would admit her patients. Finally she was forced to open her own small clinic. And four years later she <u>founded</u> her own hospital. She named it the New York <u>Infirmary</u> for Women and Children. At this point in time her work and her life were much happier.

Because of Elizabeth's <u>pioneer</u> efforts, women could now enter some medical schools. Her own sister, Emily Blackwell, and others were accepted at Western Reserve Medical School in Ohio without question. After graduation, two of these women – Emily Blackwell and Marie Sackrzenska – decided to help Dr. Blackwell found a women's medical school. Their college was the first to require a four-year course of study rather than just two. This, of course, is now common educational practice.

Elizabeth could reflect that she had come a long way since her humble beginnings. She was born in Bristol, England. When she was 11, the Blackwells came to this country. They settled first in New York, then moved to Ohio. Suddenly her father died. There were nine children in the Blackwell family. There was simply no money. Elizabeth and two sisters, Anna and Marion, started a small school in their home. This somehow kept a roof over the family's head. Later on several of her brothers became business men. They were then able to help support the family and free Elizabeth to start college.

Not long before her 50th birthday, Elizabeth Blackwell decided to go back to the land of her birth. She wrote, "The early pioneer work in the United States is ended. Throughout the Northern section of the country the free and equal entrance of women into the profession of medicine is secure." She put her sister Emily in charge of the clinic and the college and moved to London. Here she found there was still work to be done. She drew on past experience to found the London School of Medicine. She lived in England for the rest of her long life. She spent her time and a great deal of energy working on causes that were important to her. Some of these were medical education for women, preventive medicine, personal health and <u>hygiene</u>, and sex education. She died in 1910 at the age of 89. The stone at the head of her grave reads:

In loving memory of Elizabeth Blackwell, M.D. – born at Bristol, 3rd February 1821, died at Hastings 31st May, 1910. The first woman of modern times to graduate in medicine (1849) and the first to be placed on the British Medical Register (1859).

How much the women of today who wish to enter the field of medicine owe to Elizabeth Blackwell! There is <u>virtually</u> no school of medicine that denies them entry here and most other countries of the world. In Philadelphia no door was open to Elizabeth. Now that city is proud of its Women's Medical College, one of the finest schools of its kind in the country. Women are now judged on the same merits as men. They stand or fall on their own <u>scholastic</u> records. You will find them in hospitals and in private offices. You will find them in clinics and in laboratories. There is no special field of medicine which they have not entered: <u>anesthesiology</u>, <u>ophthamology</u>, <u>radiology</u>, surgery, dentistry, <u>veterinary</u> medicine, and many more. And they all owe a debt of gratitude to Elizabeth Blackwell, who bravely and stubbornly broke down the <u>barricades</u>.

On a separate sheet of paper list all the underlined words in the story about Elizabeth Blackwell. Find them in the vocabulary section beginning on page 67. Review their meaning and pronunciation. Choose any four and write a sentence for each one.

ELIZABETH BLACKWELL
Configurations

LESSON NO. 1

Draw a line from the word to the pattern (configuration) that matches it. Then print the word in the space.

school

college

doctor

study

practice

surgery

health

clinic

hospital

ELIZABETH BLACKWELL
Activities

LESSON NO. 2

In Class

1. Write a letter to your local American Medical Association. Ask if they know of anyone who could come to your class and discuss how many years it takes to become a doctor.

2. Discussion: Why do you suppose men were so against a woman's becoming a doctor? Were their reasons good or bad?

3. Discussion: Is there any profession or trade today that does not admit women?

At Home

1. Get out the telephone directory. Count the doctors in your town or city.

   How many are men? _____ How many are women? _____

2. Study a television programming schedule for a week. Try to find one about a woman doctor. Watch it. Write a paragraph about it.

At the Library

1. Investigate to make sure that all medical schools in this country now admit women.

2. Pick a specialty in medicine and find at least one article about it. Make an oral report to the class on this article.

LOUIS PASTEUR
The Man in the Laboratory

The Problem

Run! Run! Mad dog! Such a shout sent everyone dashing for cover. Before 1885 a bite from a <u>rabid</u> animal meant certain death. And it was a horrible one. Not only dogs got <u>rabies</u>. Cats, skunks, and other small animals could also be infected and would bite anyone who came near. The bitten victim began to suffer almost at once. First the section around the bite grew very painful. The victim seemed sad and depressed. Next the throat became thickly coated with a <u>mucus</u>. The victim could not swallow even though he might be screaming for water. Loud, harsh coughing did not clear the throat. Finally violent spasms shook the victim's body. And then death. It was an awful thing to watch.

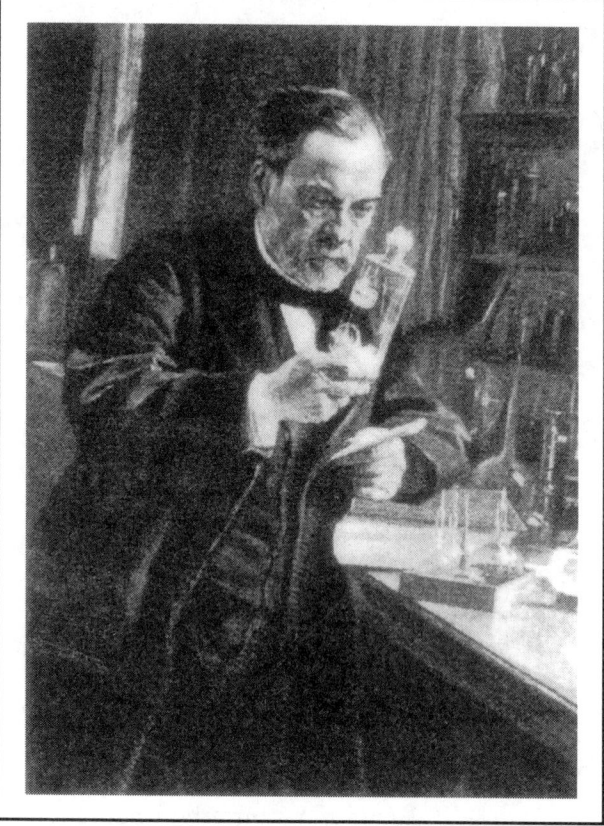

. . . Pictorial History Research

The Solution

Even today most people think that Louis Pasteur was a doctor. He was not. He was first a chemist. Then he became a <u>bacteriologist</u>. A bacteriologist is someone who studies tiny organisms called <u>bacteria</u>. There can be good and bad bacteria. For example, good bacteria help to make wine and some cheeses. Bad bacteria cause people to get sick. Pasteur was interested in both kinds of bacteria. The world is indeed lucky that this field held such interest for him.

Pasteur was born in France in 1822. When he was 16, he was sent to a school in Paris. Here he was to study and get ready for college entrance exams. However, he became so homesick that his father had to come and get him and take him home.

In time he overcame his homesickness. Then he was able to attend several fine colleges. The finest of these was the Sorbonne in Paris. After years of study he received the high degree of doctor of science. This started him on his long and <u>distinguished</u> career.

Pasteur was a hard worker all of his life. In fact, today we would call him a "workaholic." One time he wrote home, "Three things – <u>will</u>, work, and success – between them will fill a man's life." People who knew him felt that of the three, "work" was the most important to Pasteur. When he fell in love with a young French woman, he could not keep from worrying.

Would marriage keep him from his work? He even wrote the young woman a note telling her of his fears. He must have overcome them – just as he did homesickness – because they did indeed marry. And is so often the case, Marie turned out to be the perfect wife for a dedicated scientist. She felt that her husband's work should come before everything – even his family. Some time after their marriage, Pasteur became gravely ill. In spite of his wife's good care, the illness was followed by paralysis. It took many months before he was well enough to return to work.

What made Pasteur great? It may well have been his boundless curiosity. Also, he seemed willing and able to tackle any new challenge. In 1854 he was given the post of dean at a science facility at Lille. Lille was surrounded by vineyards. The making and selling of wine was very important to the people there. However, they often had problems with wine that had turned sour. Why was this happening, the people wanted to know. Pasteur set to work in his lab. The wine was growing sour, he came to believe, because a certain kind of bacteria was present. Get rid of the bacteria. No more sour wine! He saved millions of dollars for the French government. And the people of Lille were grateful forever.

It followed then that what kept wine from getting sour would also work with milk. Pasteur learned that heating liquids to a certain temperature killed bacteria. Milk heated to 140 degrees is safe. Once this process was begun, people no longer got sick from drinking milk. We call this process pasteurization.

His next challenge was a bunch of sick silkworms in the south of France. Silk was big business in France. It was one of the country's most profitable industries. And it was about to be wrecked by the ailing silkworms. No one knew what to do. Pasteur spent three years in his lab. He found that two diseases were causing the worms to get sick. And he also found a way to prevent them. He may well have saved the entire silkworm industry.

His next subjects were sheep and cattle. In France these flocks were dying by the hundreds. The cause was a disease called anthrax. By this time Pasteur had heard of the work of the Englishman Edward Jenner. He copied Jenner by taking a weak form of the anthrax bacteria and making it into a vaccine. This was then injected into the animals. They became sick quickly but it was only a mild attack. From then on they were immune to the dreaded anthrax.

When chickens in France got cholera, Pasteur used the same technique. And it worked! There seemed nothing to which he was not willing to turn his attention and his genius.

Then came his greatest triumph! French people were dying of rabies, especially in the heat of the summer. Back to his lab went Pasteur. Once again he mixed up a vaccine, this time to fight rabies. The vaccine was used for the first time on a boy who had been bitten by a mad dog. The youngster did not get rabies! A few months later the vaccine was used on a shepherd. This man also stayed well. It is important for us to remember that these young people and their families showed a great deal of courage. They were taking part in something new, something so dangerous that it might have ended in death. All the French people honored them. In fact, there is a fine statue of the brave young shepherd on the grounds of the Pasteur Institute in Paris.

The Pasteur Institute opened its doors in November of 1888. Many honors had come to Pasteur by that time. But it is likely that having an institute named after him in his <u>native</u> land meant the most to him.

Pasteur kept working until at last his health failed. The paralysis that had struck 27 years earlier returned. His family and friends were with him when he slipped away from life one sunny afternoon in autumn, 1895.

On a separate sheet of paper list all the underlined words in the story about Louis Pasteur. Find them in the vocabulary section beginning on page 67. Review their meaning and pronunciation. Choose any four and write a sentence for each one.

LOUIS PASTEUR
Word Meanings

LESSON NO. 1

The 12 words listed below were all taken from the story about Louis Pasteur. Each one has at least two distinctly different meanings. Try to write down as many meanings as you can before using the dictionary.

1. swallow

2. clear

3. kind

4. fine

5. felt

6. case

7. well

8. safe

9. form

10. watch

11. note

12. post

LOUIS PASTEUR
Activities

LESSON NO. 2

In Class

1. Discussion: Which of Pasteur's discoveries was the most important? Why?

2. Discussion: How many members of the class have ever been bitten by any kind of animal? How was it discovered that the animal was not rabid? What would class members do if an alarm was sounded that there was a rabid dog in the school yard?

At Home

1. Pretend you are a newspaper reporter. You have just learned that Louis Pasteur has found a vaccine to prevent rabies. Write a headline for an article about this.

2. Now write the article.

At the Library

1. Look up the treatment one must undergo if bitten by a rabid animal. Has this changed since the time of Pasteur? If so, how?

2. Investigate to see if France is still a leader in the production of pure silk. What other countries use silkworms for this industry?

JOSEPH LISTER
Germ Killer

The Problem

"Be sure to wash your hands before you sit down for lunch!" How many times have we all heard that? Well! Children who lived before the mid-1800's did not hear it. This was because until that time no one had been aware of germs. No one knew about the terrible damage they could do to lives.

The Solution

It took a very <u>curious</u> fellow to discover the role that germs play in the practice of medicine. His name was Joseph Lister. Lister was an Englishman. He was educated in Quaker schools as a youth. Later he went to <u>University</u> <u>College</u> Hospital for his medical studies. These were important days in medical history. For example, while a medical student, Lister was lucky. He was allowed to

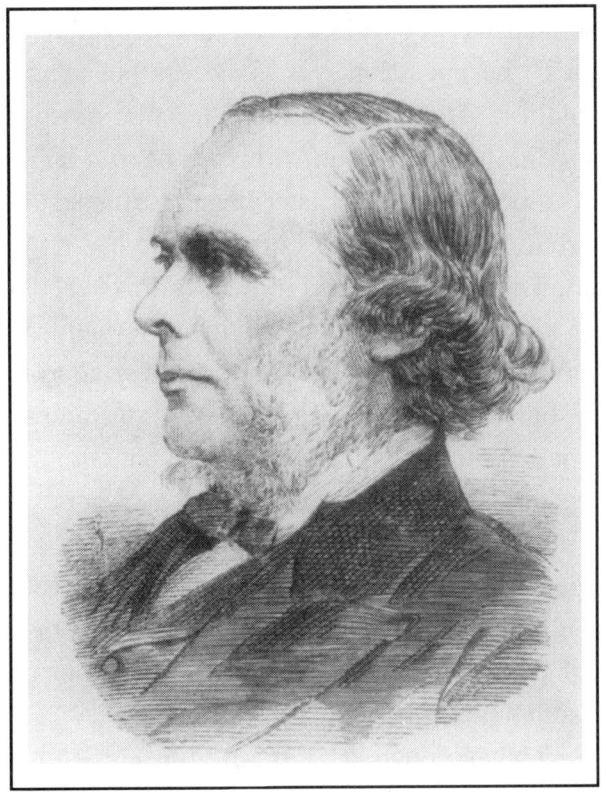

. . . North Wind Picture Archives

watch the first operation in England when the patient had been "put to sleep" by the use of <u>ether</u>. This is a fairly routine course of action now. It was an enormous breakthrough in 1852.

Lister decided he wanted to become a surgeon. He heard about Dr. James Syme. Dr. Syme was on staff at the Royal <u>Infirmary</u> in Edinburgh, Scotland. He was thought to be the leading surgeon in all of Europe. Lister went to Edinburgh. He planned to stay a month and ended up staying seven years! Dr. Syme quickly saw the young doctor's unusual <u>dedication</u> and abilities. Before long Lister had the great honor to be appointed Syme's house surgeon. In this position he had 12 assistants. A year later he was given the post of Assistant Surgeon.

Relations between the famous Dr. Syme and the young English doctor were more than just doctor to student. As a matter of fact, in 1856 Lister married Agnes Syme. She was his chief's eldest daughter. He could not have made a better choice. Throughout history successful men have often had a devoted wife in the background. Agnes Lister was a perfect example of this. She gave him all of her time and attention. When he began his practice in surgery, she ran his office. She acted as both secretary and research assistant. They were to be together for 40 years.

At first Lister's surgical practice was quite small. In fact, Agnes once laughed and referred to "Poor Joseph and his one patient." However, things suddenly took a turn for the better. Lister was appointed head of the department of clinical surgery at the Glasgow Royal <u>Infirmary</u>.

Surgical techniques in those days were quite well advanced. Men like Syme and Lister operated with confidence. Technically their skills were very good. The problem was that many times "the operation was a success but the patient died." Why? No one seemed to be able to explain it. The evidence indicated that most <u>post-operative</u> patients died from infection. Again, why did infection set in with such heartbreaking <u>regularity</u>?

About this time Lister began to suspect that perhaps something in the air might be causing infections. Just what this might be he had no idea. But he felt it was worthy of careful investigation. Then, he happened to hear of Pasteur's work with wine. Pasteur had discovered that a certain kind of <u>bacteria</u> caused wine to <u>ferment</u>. Lister thought about this long and hard. It seemed a bit of a stretch but if bacteria caused wine to ferment, what might it do to <u>post-surgical</u> wounds? The only way to prove this was to find some agent that would kill bacteria. However, it had to be something that would not harm the patient.

In his search Lister heard of a chemist in Manchester. This man had used <u>carbolic acid</u> to disinfect sewage. Might this work on the surgical wounds of human beings? Lister began a series of experiments. He kept on until he found just how much to dilute carbolic acid so that it would kill germs but would not harm patients. He went a step further. He <u>reasoned</u> that it would probably be wise to dip surgical instruments in carbolic acid as well. Now it was time for a test on a patient.

The patient was a man who had broken his leg in several places. It required skilled, <u>complicated</u> surgery. This was the kind of operation that was almost always followed by infection and then, <u>tragically</u>, <u>amputation</u>, if not death. Lister drew on his great skill to repair the damaged leg. Then he could only sit back and wait. Day after day went by and no infection! The patient did not have to undergo the terror of an amputation. He had his leg – and his life!

Lister then felt free to try this new method on other patients. In 1867 he published a report of his first cases. The report told how he had operated on eleven patients and had used the carbolic acid treatment. Of the eleven, one died. One required amputation. The others all lived full and rich lives. He spent two more years proving and <u>perfecting</u> his method. Then and only then did he feel it was safe to announce his discovery. His findings appeared in the *British Medical Journal*. They quickly spread throughout the world of medicine.

He made his treatment even simpler to use. He invented the carbolic spray. At first surgical wounds were sprayed by hand. Then a pump was developed, and finally a machine did the job. The carbolic spray was found in every operating room for the next 20 years. It made use of carbolic acid in post-operative patients much easier.

In 1897 Joseph Lister became Lord Lister. In 1903 England further honored him by using his name for one of the finest research centers in the country. They called it the Lister <u>Institute</u> of

Preventive Medicine. He died in 1912 at the age of 85. A friend in the Royal College of Surgeons wrote:

> His gentle nature, _imperturbable_ temper, resolute _will_, indifference to ridicule, and tolerance of hostile criticism, combined to make him one of the noblest of men. His work will last for all time; humanity will bless him evermore and his fame will be _immortal_.

———————————————

On a separate sheet of paper list all the underlined words in the story about Joseph Lister. Find them in the vocabulary section beginning on page 67. Review their meaning and pronunciation. Choose any four and write a sentence for each one.

JOSEPH LISTER
Break the Code

LESSON NO. 1

The following questions are in code. Break the code by changing each letter to the one that precedes it in the alphabet. Then write your one or two-word answer in the same code.

1. XIBU XBT MJTUFS'T TQFDJBMUZ?

   _____

   _____

2. XIBU XBT MJTUFS'T XJGF'T OBNF?

   _____

   _____

3. JO XIBU TDPUUJTI DJUZ EJE MJTUFS QSBDUJDF?

   _____

   _____

4. XIBU DBVTFE JOGFDUJPO BGUFS PQFSBUJPOT?

   _____

   _____

5. XIBU XBT VTFE UP QVU QBUJFOUT UP TMFFQ?

   _____

   _____

6. XIBU MJRVJE XBT QBTUFVS XPSLJOH PO?

   _____

   _____

7. XIBU EJTJOGFDUBOU EJE MJTUFS VTF?

   _____

   _____

8. XIBU DPNNFSDJBM QSPEVDU VTFT MJTUFS'T OBNF?

   _____

   _____

JOSEPH LISTER
Activities

LESSON NO. 2

In Class

1. Lister used some of Pasteur's findings in his work. Make up a dialogue that might have taken place between the two men should they have met.

2. Consult a science text and see if you can find a simple experiment for growing bacteria in the classroom.

At Home

1. Read the labels on 4 liquids used at your house for cleaning. List the names of any that use the word "germ."

2. Look through magazines and find 4 ads for toothpaste, mouthwash, or other household product that mention "germ free" or "disinfectant."

At the Library

1. Lister attended Quaker schools as a youth. Find out all you can about the Quaker movement in England and the United States.

2. Look up carbolic acid. Is it dangerous? What is it used for today?

MARIA MONTESSORI
Doctor - Teacher - Pioneer

The Problem

Be glad that you did not have to go to school in the 19th Century! Schools were not the lively, colorful places they are now. The buildings were dark and gloomy. Punishment was harsh and frequent. Teachers were not well trained. And the methods! Students were forced to memorize everything. There was little art, little music, little chance for young minds to ask questions and to grow. Maria Montessori compared Italian schools to prisons, and she was right!

The Solution

Maria Montessori was born in 1870 in Eastern Italy. She was an only child. The one thing Maria was sure that she did *not* want to be was a teacher. What *did* she want to be? She was not sure. Perhaps an <u>engineer</u>. It was

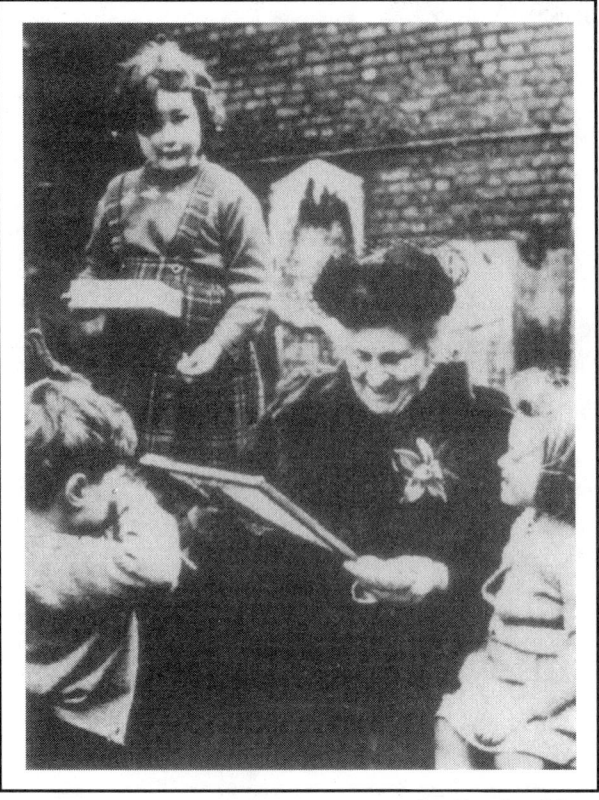

. . . San Francisco Library

an odd choice for a girl. So Maria had to go to a boys' high school. Several other girls were there, too. During recess all the girls were kept in a room to keep them away from the boys.

After high school, Maria went to a <u>technical</u> school. Somehow it was not what she had thought it would be. So she changed her mind. She decided she wanted to become a doctor. Her father was against it and tried to talk her out of it. But her mother <u>encouraged</u> the change in career plans.

Maria entered medical school. Her father laid down certain rules that would seem strange to us today. He insisted that someone walk with her to and from school each day. Also, she had to sit apart from the male students in the <u>lecture</u> halls. As a matter of fact, the farther she could get away from them, the better! They were not friendly. They said rude things to her. They shook her desk when she was trying to write. They shut her out of student life as much as possible.

Another problem was the study of the human skeleton. To do this, students had to <u>dissect</u> human bodies and organs. Of course, Maria was not allowed to work alongside the male students. Instead she had to return to the lab at night when everyone else had gone home. It must have been a creepy place – skeletons, skulls, hearts and livers and other organs in jars on shelves.

During these years and perhaps because of the treatment of the male students, Maria grew interested in the rights of women. Not many of them were able to choose a career as she had done. She kept this interest for the rest of her life.

It took six years but finally Maria Montessori became the first woman doctor in Italy. She could, of course, treat only women and children. And this led to her early interest in children who were <u>mentally retarded</u>. In those days it was thought in error that mentally retarded children could not be taught anything but the most simple, basic tasks. They led sad lives – no toys or books or music. It was felt that they were not worth taking the time or trouble to try to teach. Dr. Montessori did not agree. She began to develop new methods and new materials. She believed that children needed to use all their senses in order to learn – sight, hearing, touch, smell. She believed that classrooms should be light, cheerful, orderly. She believed that children should be allowed to experiment with shapes and <u>textures</u> and weights.

She also believed that good health and a good diet were important and – a totally new thought – children really *wanted* to learn. If they were given the right materials and the right opportunities and the right experiences, they would, indeed, learn.

After a while she came up with a new thought. If this approach worked so well with the mentally retarded, why not use it with <u>normal</u> children? And, of course she was right!

The next step was to train young teachers to use her methods. Her classes quickly grew popular as she showed teachers just how joyful teaching could be. At the same time she started a school for young Italian children. It was called *Casa dei Bambini* (House of Children). This grew to a second school. And then to other schools as more and more parents demanded that their children be taught with Montessori methods. Since she could not train all the teachers in the world – or even in Italy – she sat down and wrote a book. It was called *The Montessori Method*. Later it was <u>translated</u> into more than 20 languages. People from other countries came to study with her. Soon there were Montessori method schools in England, the United States, India, China, Mexico, and a number of other countries. In Russia the <u>tsar</u> opened a Montessori school in his palace. His own children went to it along with children of members of his court.

Dr. Montessori was invited to speak all over the world. The time had come when she had to give up her medical practice in favor of her other interests. One of her most successful tours took place in the United States. It should be remembered that in those days there was no TV and very little radio. When a well-known speaker came to town, the hall was usually packed. Maria Montessori was in demand because she had two topics to discuss. The first, of course, was education. The second had to do with her long-held interest in the rights of women, rights which were few and far between in those days. It seems hard to believe that some scientists thought that women's brains were inferior to men's. And most of the best schools in higher education still would not admit women. Montessori took a strong stand against such <u>inequalities</u>.

The Montessori method did have some problems. Dr. Montessori could not visit every school to be sure they were meeting her standards. This was especially true in times of war. Some teachers, who had studied with her, accepted her ideas without question; others wanted to add their own ideas to the method. So from time to time the two groups quarreled.

When she was 81, Dr. Montessori was planning a trip to Africa. Then she suffered a stroke and died in 1952. Young people reading the story of her life may not know it but their lives have most likely been touched by Maria Montessori. She gave the world a better understanding of how children grow and learn. Her methods can be found in bright classrooms where the desks and chairs are child-sized. Where the books and materials are fascinating and challenging. Where there is art and music and hands-on materials. Where students are urged to explore and experiment. Where teachers take time to listen.

The memory of Maria Montessori will be forever honored in schools, large and small, all over the world.

———————————

On a separate sheet of paper list all the underlined words in the story about Maria Montessori. Find them in the vocabulary section beginning on page 67. Review their meaning and pronunciation. Choose any four and write a sentence for each one.

MARIA MONTESSORI
Synonyms, Antonyms, Homonyms

LESSON NO. 1

All of the words in the left-hand columns come from the story about Maria Montessori.

1. Draw a line to the word that means the same or almost the same. The first one has been done for you.

prison	castle
people	feel
strange	certain
palace	jail
touch	woman
little	impolite
sure	belief
female	odd
rude	small
thought	persons

2. Draw a line to the word that means the opposite. The first one has been done for you.

higher	exit
enter	worst
farther	dull
strong	small
best	together
true	false
bright	lower
large	end
apart	weak
start	nearer

1. Draw a line to the word that has the same sound but a different meaning. The first one has been done for you.

right	mail
not	wait
male	knot
days	knight
new	four
weight	write
one	witch
night	knew
for	won
which	daze

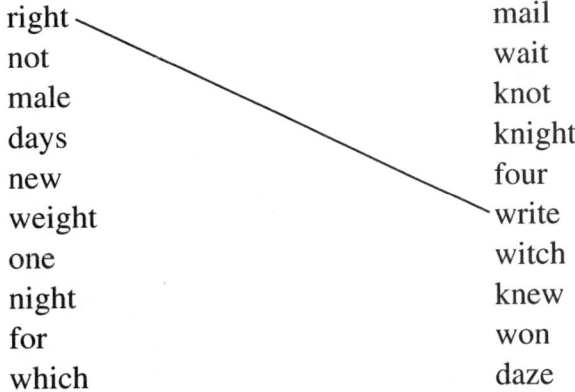

MARIA MONTESSORI
Activities

LESSON NO. 2

In Class

1. Write a letter to a Montessori school in your town or city. Request that someone from this school visit your class to talk about the Montessori method.

2. Write a paragraph about how it must have been for Maria to return to the lab alone at night. Make it sound creepy and spooky with lots of shadows and strange noises.

At Home

1. Write a description of what you think would make a perfect classroom. Include a floor plan if you wish.

2. Prepare a lesson plan for very young children that includes some of Dr. Montessori's ideas.

At the Library

1. Check out a book written about Maria Montessori (or a book that has a chapter about her). Take turns reading it aloud in class, a little each day.

2. Write a review of that book. Did you like it? Why? Why not? Do you agree with Dr. Montessori's methods? Why? Why not?

ALBERT SCHWEITZER
Man for All Seasons

The Problem

In the 1800's many missionaries had gone to Africa. They were sent by churches all over the world to help the natives of Africa in any way they could. There was much that they could and did do. But their skills were few when it came to the massive medical need. Most missionaries knew little more than the basic remedy of keeping wounds clean. Much more knowledge and skill were needed. There were few doctors, if any, in certain regions. And there were no hospitals. Disease that should have been stopped, spread. Lives that could have been saved were lost.

The Solution

All of this changed when a man named Albert Schweitzer picked up a magazine one evening. In it he read an article titled "The Needs

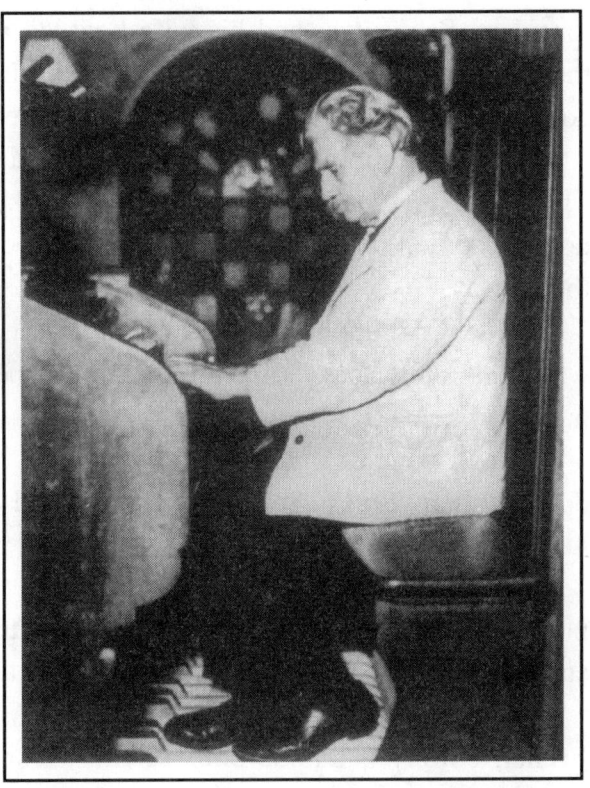

. . . Underwood Photo Archives

of the Congo Mission." He took a <u>vow</u> then and there that he would go to Africa. In a way it was a strange vow. Before he was 30 Schweitzer had become a famous man. He seemed to have many interests. One was the study of religion. He preached at local churches. He wrote books about his deep feelings. Another interest was music. He was a fine organist. He had studied the organ so well that he could actually build one from parts. He also wrote about organ music and the men who composed it.

Here was a man with a full rich life. He had friends, family, fame, his work. But on the spur of the moment he decided to give it all up. Another part of his vow caused everyone to gasp. He said that the Congo needed doctors. So he would become a doctor. It took him seven years!

Medical school was long and difficult for him. For one thing he did not have much money. He paid for his schooling and his living expenses by giving organ concerts. One spring he went to Paris to learn as much as he could about <u>tropical</u> diseases. He knew he would find many of these in the Congo. He felt he needed to know how to treat them.

One of his friends was named Helene Bresslau. In fact, she was the daughter of one of his teachers. Schweitzer used to visit her home to hold long discussions with her father. Helene knew that Schweitzer was determined to go to Africa as soon as he became a doctor. She had fallen in love with him so she wanted to go with him. She enrolled in a nursing school. This way she would be helpful as an assistant in his work in Africa. They were married in 1912. The honeymoon was a trip to Berlin to learn even more about tropical diseases.

The final <u>hurdle</u> was money. Somehow Schweitzer was able to beg or borrow enough money to pay for the trip. Also, he filled 70 packing cases with medical supplies. A doctor at long last, Schweitzer and his wife boarded a small steamer for a hard journey. At Port Gentil they transferred to a riverboat. The trip through the jungle to their new home was hot, with few comforts. After only a few days – but what seemed much longer – they reached Lambaréné.

The first glimpse of Lambaréné was a shock. Schweitzer had been promised a hospital. There was none. He was given a filthy chicken house in which to see patients. His supplies had not yet come. Yet word had spread. Sick people showed up by the hundreds. He had to send them away.

When his supplies reached him at last, he began treating patients on his front porch. Helene was at his side. Heavy rains forced him to operate in the chicken house. It was clear that a hospital had to be built as soon as possible.

Finally one of the riverboats unloaded building supplies. No one seemed to know what to do with them. So Dr. Schweitzer had to add the job of seeing the hospital was built properly to his heavy medical duties.

It took time but the Africans did come to know that the white doctor's medicine was more powerful than the witch doctor's. Some of the native beliefs amazed him. He could not understand why newborn babies were painted white. This was to ward off evil spirits, he was told.

The Schweitzers were German. When World War I broke out in 1914, they were living in a French colony – Lambaréné. To the French at that time, any German was an enemy. The Schweitzers were sent to prison camps in France. Here they had to stay until the war's end. Conditions in the camps were unhealthy. By the time they were released, Dr. Schweitzer was not well. He had been deeply saddened by his mother's death. And the ruined cities left by the war depressed him.

The birth of a daughter helped restore his good spirits. But now Helene's health was not good. So he had to return to Lambaréné alone. He found his hospital in a <u>shambles</u> and set to work at once to rebuild it. At long last other doctors and nurses began to join him. Later a <u>site</u> for a new hospital was chosen. Dr. Schweitzer had to spend much of his time raising money to build it. Fundraising was easier now. Schweitzer's work was known all over the world. People were eager to help. Visitors came from many countries. More trained staff people arrived to help lighten the load.

Again war clouds began to gather. Dr. Schweitzer made another vow. This time he said he would never set foot in Germany again until the Nazis were defeated. He kept his word. Helene was stronger and able to return to Lambaréné. That same year a gift of supplies arrived from the United States just when Schweitzer thought he was going to have to close the hospital. The work went on.

After World War II ended, Schweitzer spent time writing books and articles. He gave many speeches. He was fighting as best he could against the spread of <u>nuclear</u> weapons. During this time he received many honors. By far the highest was the Nobel Peace Prize in 1953. He did not go to Sweden to accept the prize. There was too much work to be done in the Congo. But he spent the prize money on the hospital.

Four years later Helene died in Switzerland. Dr. Schweitzer, sad and old, kept on with his work at Lambaréné. He no longer took care of patients. But there was still much to be done if the hospital was to keep its record for excellent care. He died quietly at age 90 one September evening. On all lists of the ten greatest men who ever lived, you are sure to find the name of Albert Schweitzer somewhere near the top.

On a separate sheet of paper list all the underlined words in the story about Albert Schweitzer. Find them in the vocabulary section beginning on page 67. Review their meaning and pronunciation. Choose any four and write a sentence for each one.

ALBERT SCHWEITZER
Categories

LESSON NO. 1

Most of the words below come from the story about Albert Schweitzer. Underline the word in each line that doesn't belong.

1.	piano	organ	flute	pencil
2.	word	friend	pal	chum
3.	riverboat	lifeboat	books	rowboat
4.	trip	patients	voyage	journey
5.	duties	hundreds	thousands	millions
6.	shambles	jumble	mess	gift
7.	prize	award	honor	camp
8.	Germany	France	Detroit	Sweden
9.	years	religion	months	days
10.	age	September	June	February
11.	jungle	desert	money	forest
12.	Africans	home	Americans	Germans
13.	work	rain	hail	snow
14.	white	purple	yellow	baby
15.	disease	gift	illness	sickness
16.	doctor	teacher	building	lawyer
17.	list	evening	morning	afternoon
18.	magazine	book	fame	newspaper
19.	promise	pledge	vow	tropical
20.	spring	expense	winter	summer

ALBERT SCHWEITZER
Activities

LESSON NO. 2

In Class

1. Write a paragraph about how it might feel to be interned in a prisoner of war camp.

2. Write a paragraph either for or against the use of nuclear weapons.

At Home

1. List 5 reasons why you would like to be a missionary.

    or

2. List 5 reasons why you would not like to be a missionary.

At the Library

1. One of the composers of organ music that Dr. Schweitzer wrote about was Johann Sebastian Bach. See what you can find out about him.

2. Many things have changed about the Congo since Dr. Schweitzer did his fine work there. Discover at least 5 interesting facts about it.

ALEXANDER FLEMING
Hard Work or Luck

The Problem

It wasn't so many years ago that if you grew ill with <u>strep throat</u> or <u>appendicitis</u>, you might not get well. Your family doctor knew what was wrong with you. But he or she didn't know how to cure it. The doctor most likely also knew what was causing the problem. It was <u>bacteria</u> living and growing and spreading deep in your body. But there was simply no known medicine to kill the infection.

The Solution

Enter Alexander Fleming! It was he who, almost by chance, came up with an answer to these age-old medical problems. With this single discovery, Fleming entered the ranks of the great men in medicine, the savers of lives.

Fleming was born on a farm in Scotland in 1881. He was the youngest of eight children. He

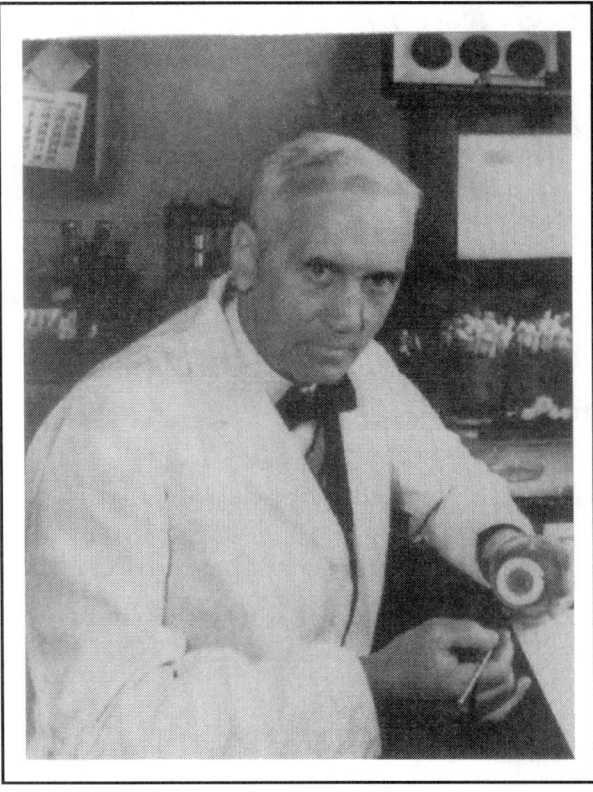

. . . Underwood Photo Archives

might have become a farmer. He loved the outdoors and life on a farm. But the farm went to his oldest brother Hugh. Instead he was sent to London. Here he lived with two other brothers and went to school. His brothers were in medical school. They wanted Fleming to study medicine, too. He was a good swimmer so he chose the medical school that had the best waterpolo team! He took part in all sports and won most of the school's prizes for good work in his studies. As soon as he completed medical school, he went to work in a lab. Here he earned more honors for his research.

World War I broke out in 1914. Fleming joined the Royal Army Medical Corp. He was sent to Boulogne in France. He could not believe the terrible conditions he found there. Buildings had been turned into grim, crowded hospitals. He saw men die of wounds that should have healed. <u>Antiseptics</u> failed to halt the <u>bacteria</u> they were supposed to get rid of. Captain Fleming never forgot the war. He went back to his lab, hoping to find something that would kill the bacteria that had caused so much illness and death. But there was a danger. He feared that anything that would kill bacteria might also harm healthy <u>tissue</u>.

It was a summer day many years later when Fleming saw something strange in his lab. He had put a batch of <u>staph</u> germs in a shallow dish. Staph germs are deadly. They can kill. Later

Fleming noticed that some mold was covering part of the staph germs in the shallow dish. This was not unusual. It often happened in the lab. But something very peculiar was going on. The area around the mold was free of staph germs. Something in the mold was killing the germs! What kind of mold was this? No one could be quite sure. It may have started from a speck of dust that floated through a window and landed on the dish of staph germs. No matter what it was, Fleming knew it had to be explored.

He found that he was able to grow that mold in his lab on bread, cheese, and fruit. It thrived in meat juices. He used mice for his experiments. First he infected them with the awful staph and strep germs. Then he gave them a dose of the mysterious mold in liquid form. Behold! The germs vanished! The mice lived!

Fleming named his discovery penicillin. He announced it in a British journal in 1929. Strangely enough, not a great deal of attention was paid to this news. In fact, some doctors and scientists did not believe it. They thought it was some kind of superstition or folklore. For ten years the power of penicillin was more or less overlooked. Part of the problem was that it was difficult to make.

Then two outstanding men became interested. Dr. Howard W. Florey held a degree in medicine. Dr. Ernst Boris Chain was a German chemist. He left his family behind when he came to work in England because he felt Hitler's power would not last long. He was wrong. His mother and sister were put to death in a German concentration camp. These two men worked together month after month trying to extract medicine from Fleming's mold. At last they got a teaspoonful of yellow-brown powder and tested it on mice.

According to some sources, penicillin was first used on a human in February 1941. The patient was a London policeman. He had a bad staph infection. His face was a mass of running sores. His fever was 105 degrees. His doctors had been using the new sulfa drugs. He did not respond. Then he was given a shot of penicillin. His fever dropped at once. But too much damage had already taken place, and he died.

Next penicillin was used on a fifteen-year-old boy. He was dangerously ill with a strep infection. He made a full recovery. Other children were treated with penicillin and got well.

Then the horrors of World War II struck! It was then that penicillin became one of the world's most important drugs. But there was a problem. England was under heavy air attack by German planes. It could not make penicillin in the great quantities that were needed. Dr. Florey flew to the United States. He took with him samples of the mold, some penicillin extract, and all of the records on the drug. The trip, of course, was very secret. The danger of being shot down by German aircraft was great.

American scientists went to work. Soon penicillin was being produced in huge vats by a number of drug companies. They all continued to search for stronger molds. One time their search was aided by an Illinois woman. She took a rotten moldy cantaloupe to one of the labs. There it was found that this mold made an extremely powerful form of penicillin. They called her "Moldy Mary."

In 1944 Fleming was knighted. It was now *Sir* Alexander Fleming. In 1945, together with Dr. Florey and Dr. Chain, he was awarded the Nobel Prize.

Once it became known that certain molds had the power to cure, many scientists began to investigate. As a result, a number of new and powerful molds were developed into "wonder" drugs that cured a wide variety of diseases. There is no doubt that Fleming changed the world of medicine. Many illnesses that once terrified because they resulted in death are now curable and not particularly frightening. The world owes much of this to Alexander Fleming.

He retired when he was 67, feeling that younger men should carry on his work. He died in his 74th year of a heart attack. His death took place just a few blocks from the lab where he had worked for so many years. In that lab today is a sealed jar. It contains Fleming's original mold from which came most of the world's supply of penicillin.

On a separate sheet of paper list all the underlined words in the story about Alexander Fleming. Find them in the vocabulary section beginning on page 67. Review their meaning and pronunciation. Choose any four and write a sentence for each one.

ALEXANDER FLEMING
Crossword Puzzle

LESSON NO. 1

Use the clues below to solve the crossword puzzle. The 20 words needed to solve the puzzle can be found in the box below the clues.

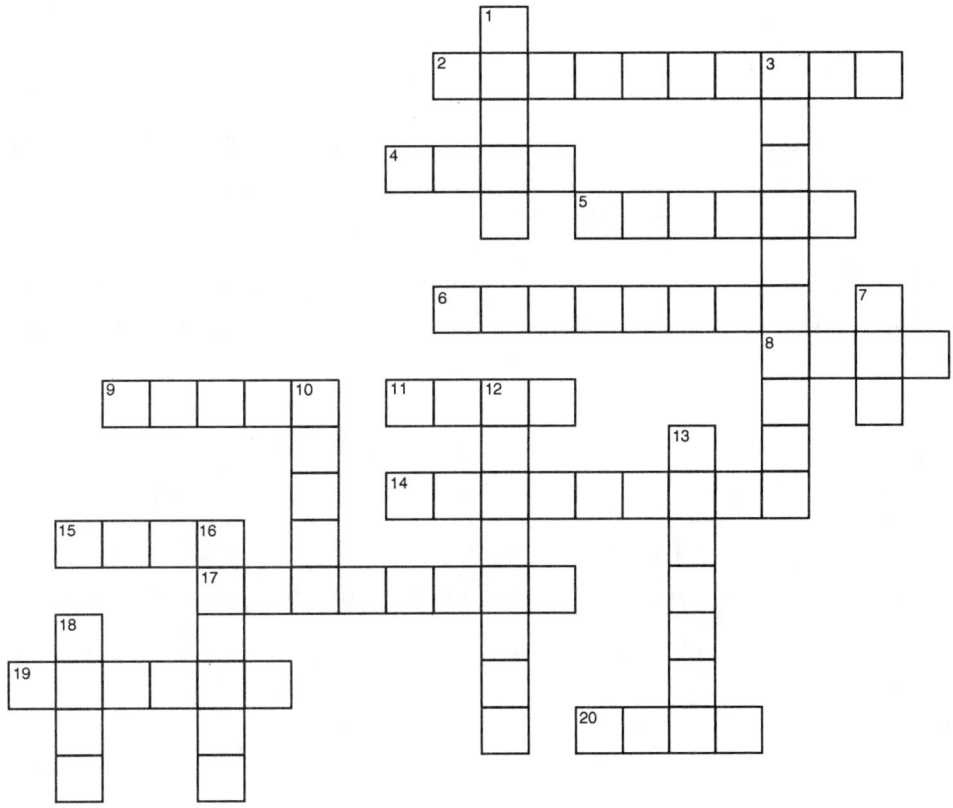

Across

2. antibiotic used to fight disease
4. land used to produce crops, livestock, etc.
5. a place where instruction is given
6. micro-organisms that may cause disease
8. a group of people working or playing together
9. an injury to the skin or flesh
11. any microscopic disease-bearing organism
14. anything learned for the first time
15. the edible flesh of animals
17. a place that provides treatment for people who are ill
19. an opening in a building to let in light
20. a fungus that produces furry growth

Down

1. the organ in the body that circulates blood
3. a room or building for scientific work or research.
7. open, armed clash between nations
10. substances used as medicine; also habit-forming narcotics
12. careful study of some field of knowledge
13. connected with the practice or study of medicine
16. the passage from the mouth to the stomach
18. a container for holding food

farm	bacteria	wound	discovery	window
penicillin	school	team	germ	meat
laboratory	medical	research	hospital	mold
heart	war	drugs	throat	dish

ALEXANDER FLEMING
Activities

LESSON NO. 2

In Class

1. Using the information obtained in #2 of the "At the Library" section below, write to three drug companies (Attention: Public Relations Department) and ask for printed material on penicillin and/or other wonder drugs.

2. Write a paragraph about any illness you or someone in your family might have had. Were wonder drugs used? How quickly did they work? Include as many details as possible.

At Home

1. Talk to someone in your family or in the neighborhood about how it was to be seriously ill before wonder drugs were discovered. Write a paragraph about what you learned.

2. Dampen a piece of bread, put it in a dark warm place, and see how long it takes to start growing mold. Take the results to school. Compare notes with classmates.

At the Library

1. Penicillin is called a wonder drug. Look up and list the names of five other wonder drugs now commonly used. Tell what they are used for.

2. Find the names and addresses of three large drug companies. Use this information for the class assignment #1 above.

ALICE HAMILTON
Danger in the Workplace

The Problem

Suppose you became ill – very ill. Your illness was caused by something at your place of work. And suppose your employer could not be held <u>responsible</u> for your condition. And your doctor really didn't know very much about this kind of illness. And there was no insurance to help you with your bills while you could not work.

The Solution

The above describes the <u>plight</u> of the worker in this country in the early 1900's. And this is what moved Alice Hamilton to enter the field of <u>industrial</u> medicine. It was a much neglected field. Until this time no one had ever been interested in it. Certainly no woman had.

In those days factory workers put in a 12-hour day and a 7-day week. There were

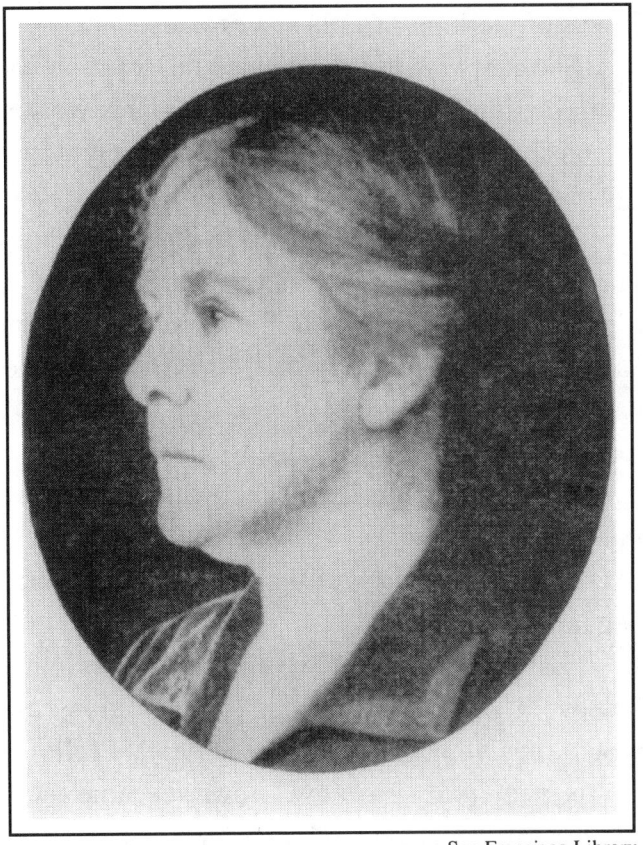

. . . San Francisco Library

no laws to protect their rights. This was some time before the strong "union movement" took place in this country when workers banded together for the first time. They formed strong unions. When conditions in the workplace did not improve, they went out on <u>strike</u>. However, when Alice Hamilton began her efforts, the factory bosses were still very much in control.

Even as a medical student Alice Hamilton had been more interested in what went on in the laboratory than in the clinic. She was fascinated by <u>bacteriology</u> and <u>pathology</u>. So much so that she wanted to skip her year as an <u>intern</u>. However, some of her teachers in medical school convinced her that she could learn much as an intern. Finally she bowed to their advice.

She completed her year as an intern at the New England Hospital for Women and Children. Then she went to Germany. There she continued the study of pathology. At the end of her studies she was asked to teach pathology at the Women's Medical School at Northwestern <u>University</u>. She took this offer because it meant she could live at Hull House in Chicago. Hull House had been founded by Jane Addams years earlier. It was a place where poor immigrants could go for food, medicine, legal advice, etc. Alice Hamilton lived there for more than 20 years. It was a good place for her. Throughout much of her life she stayed interested in the problems of the poor. At that time few others seemed to pay much attention to the needs of poor people.

It was most likely this concern that aimed her toward industrial medicine. Her interest grew when the governor of Illinois appointed her to a State Commission to study occupational diseases. The Commission was to look into those materials used in manufacturing that seemed to be toxic – materials such as arsenic, cyanide, brass, etc. Alice Hamilton's job was to look at the effects of working in a place where lead was present.

She first visited a white-lead factory. She had heard that the manager was a kind and caring man. She implied to him that some of his workers were being poisoned. He angrily denied any responsibility. This turned out to be a fairly typical response from factory owners and managers. But she pressed on.

The breakthrough seemed to come one day when she went to the National Lead Company. She talked to the vice-president, a man named Edward Cornish. He issued a challenge to her. He said, "Prove to me that my workers are being poisoned by working with lead, and I will do anything you want me to do." She set out to meet this challenge. It was not an easy task. She had to interview dozens of workers and their wives. She had to dig through stacks of medical records. Finally, she was able to prove that there were 22 cases of severe lead poisoning in Mr. Cornish's plant. He was shocked but he was a man of his word. He lived up to his promise. He put protective devices in all of his plants in the Chicago area at once. He hired doctors to watch over the health and well-being of his workers. He set a standard that other factory owners began to follow.

Just one year after the State Commission published its report, a new law was passed in Illinois. This law said that if job conditions caused a worker to be hurt or to become ill, he would receive payments. State after state followed the example set by Illinois. Soon workmen's compensation, as it is now known, became the law of the land. Even better, factory conditions were greatly changed and improved.

In a sense, this was only the start of Alice Hamilton's contributions. She looked into the toxic working conditions of a number of other industries. She made several trips to Europe as a delegate to the International Congresses for Occupational Diseases. In 1924 she was honored to be named a member of the Health Committee of the League of Nations. (The League was the international governing body that was formed after World War I. It, however, was never so effective as the United Nations, the international governing body that was formed after World War II.) She was even invited to inspect factories in Russia at a time when that huge country was not friendly to foreigners.

One day there came an unexpected honor. She was the first woman doctor to be asked to join the faculty of the Harvard Medical School. What made this astonishing was the fact that, at that time, Harvard did not yet accept women into its medical school.

In her autobiography, *Exploring the Dangerous Trades*, Dr. Hamilton wrote:

Thirty-two years ago in 1910, I went as a pioneer into a new unexplored field of American medicine, the field of industrial disease. This book is a record of what I found there, of the changes that have taken place through the years that have *followed, and of what still remains to be done before we can say that the wilderness has been conquered and the country completely <u>civilized</u>.*

Alice Hamilton was a fearless <u>liberal</u> with great strength and courage whose cause was a just one. She was, as she says, a <u>pioneer</u> in medicine. It can truthfully be said that because of her work, the world is a better place for all workers.

On a separate sheet of paper list all the underlined words in the story about Alice Hamilton. Find them in the vocabulary section beginning on page 67. Review their meaning and pronunciation. Choose any four and write a sentence for each one.

ALICE HAMILTON
Word Scramble

LESSON NO. 1

Unscramble the letters to form words from the story about Alice Hamilton. Write the words in the space to the right.

1. E W K E   W _ _ _
2. T E N N R I   I _ _ _ _ _
3. O U I N N   U _ _ _ _
4. D E L A   L _ _ _
5. C O I T X   T _ _ _ _
6. G R E N A M A   M _ _ _ _ _ _
7. R E N E P O I   P _ _ _ _ _ _
8. I R P T   T _ _ _
9. T R O O C D   D _ _ _ _ _
10. D E L I F   F _ _ _ _
11. S A B R S   B _ _ _ _
12. S P O O N I   P _ _ _ _ _
13. W O R R E K   W _ _ _ _ _
14. T R Y C O A F   F _ _ _ _ _ _
15. S O B S   B _ _ _
16. B L O R E M P   P _ _ _ _ _ _
17. N P T L A   P _ _ _ _
18. D R O W   W _ _ _
19. S C A R I E N   A _ _ _ _ _ _
20. N E Z O D   D _ _ _ _

48

ALICE HAMILTON
Activities

LESSON NO. 2

In Class

1. Write a paragraph about why the Child Labor Laws and other laws that affect conditions in factories are a good idea.

2. Act out a dialogue between Alice Hamilton and a factory manager when she wants conditions changed and improved, and the factory manager refuses to believe there is any danger to his workers.

At Home

1. List 4 reasons why you would like to work in a factory that makes jelly beans.

   or

2. List 4 reasons why you would not like to work in a factory that makes jelly beans.

At the Library

1. Look up conditions in American and English factories in the 18th and 19th centuries when children were hired to work in factories.

2. Learn all you can about the union movement in this country – when it began, why it was needed, etc.

HELEN BROOKE TAUSSIG
Doctor with a Heart

The Problem

Until the middle of the 20th Century, there were a number of newly-born infants who quickly developed a problem with oxygen. They were called "blue babies." This was because without enough oxygen in the blood stream, the skin tended to take on a bluish hue. These babies usually died. Doctors and researchers were quite sure they knew what caused the condition. But no one seemed to know what to do about it.

Experts agreed that a blue baby had a defect in its heart. In fact, it was most often a mix of more than one defect – sometimes as many as four. If the child did not die at birth, it seldom lived longer than a few years.

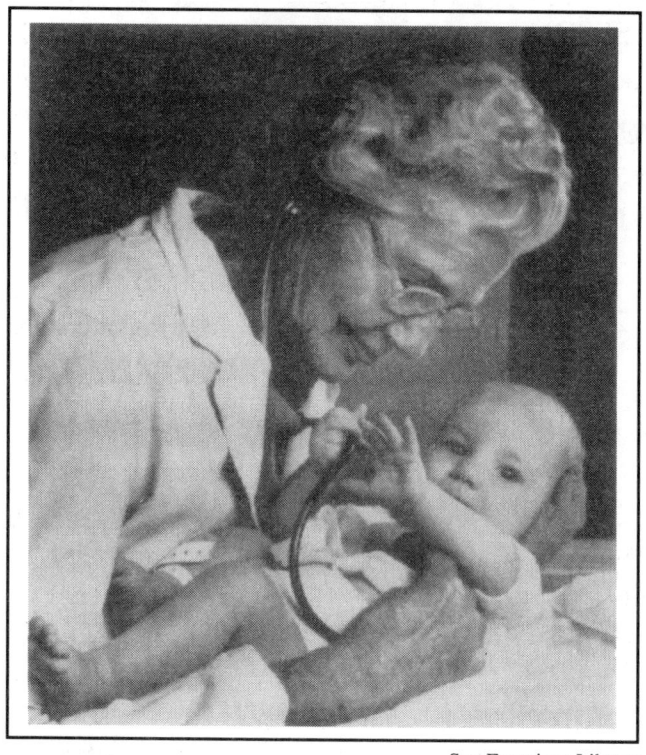

. . . San Francisco Library

The Solution

One would think that a surgeon would be needed to solve the "blue baby" problem. But it did not! Instead the answer came from a woman doctor who was not a surgeon. Not only that, Dr. Helen Taussig was dyslexic and had a severe hearing problem. She could not hear a heart beat through a stethoscope. Instead she "listened" by putting her hand lightly on the chest wall of a patient.

Helen Taussig was born in 1898 in Cambridge, Massachusetts. There she grew up but went to college in California. After completing four years, she decided she would like a career in medicine. Women were still not welcomed with open arms in the field of medicine. (Harvard did not admit women to its medical school until 1945.) So she began by taking some public health courses at Harvard. Later she transferred to the School of Medicine at Boston University. Here she studied anatomy. It turned out to be an important move. One of her teachers put her to work studying the heart muscles of an ox. This began her life-long interest in cardiology.

She kept on with her medical studies at the famed Johns Hopkins medical school. On staff there was Dr. Edward Park. This man was very interested in children's heart problems (pediatric cardiology). Many of his young patients suffered from rheumatic fever. This disease often left damage to the heart. Dr. Park felt there should be a place where such children could be treated.

He founded the Lane Pediatric Cardiac Clinic for Children. In 1930 Dr. Taussig became head of that clinic. From then on many doctors sent their "blue babies" to her.

Dr. Taussig studied and traveled widely trying to find a cure for this condition in infants. She went to Canada to consult with Dr. Maude Abbott at McGill University. She learned a great deal from this heart specialist.

Finally she had an idea that might work. It consisted of a bypass that would bring blood back to the lungs. But Dr. Taussig had a problem. She was not a surgeon. So she could not test her own theory. She went to several surgeons. Would they try this new technique? They would not! At last she found a friendly ear. Dr. Alfred Blalock agreed with what she proposed. But he felt that additional research must be done first. He operated on at least 200 dogs before he felt it was safe to try the technique on a human.

The first patient was a little girl. She was only 11 months old but her condition was so bad she could live only in an oxygen tent. Medical history was made the day of that first operation. The baby lived and grew healthy. Other successful "blue baby" operations followed. Children from all over the world were brought to the Lane Clinic.

Dr. Taussig made yet another major gift to mothers and children. One day she learned from a former student that quite a large number of deformed babies were being born in Germany. Many were missing arms or legs. Dr. Taussig left for Germany at once. She spent six weeks visiting clinics. She examined babies. She learned that all of the mothers of the deformed babies had taken the same medication. It was called Contergan. Then Dr. Haussig learned something strange. None of the newborn babies of American soldiers stationed at an army base were deformed. Except one. The mother of that child had bought Contergan at a drugstore off the base. All of the other American mothers had been treated on the base by American doctors. None were given Contergan. Their babies were fine.

Dr. Haussig quickly shared her findings with Dr. Frances Kelsey. Dr. Kelsey worked at the FDA (Food and Drug Administration) in Washington, D.C. Several drug companies had asked the FDA for permission to produce and sell Contergan. Dr. Kelsey felt that it had not yet been proven that Contergan was safe. She would not give permission. She demanded better testing. The drug companies were not happy. So it is easy to imagine how relieved Dr. Kelsey was when she heard the news about Contergan from Dr. Haussig. Here were two women who almost singlehandedly prevented terrible tragedies.

Dr. Taussig stayed on at the Lane Clinic for many years. When she retired from the clinic, she went into research full time. In 1965 she became the first woman president of the American Heart Association. She was convinced that blood vessel disease (today we call it too much cholesterol) started very early in childhood. She felt that a good low-fat diet should begin in a child's first years. Today's doctors and health professionals are in full agreement with her.

Dr. Taussig continued her good work until 1986. Then, only three days short of her 88th birthday, she was backing out of her driveway to take some friends to the polls to vote. Her car was hit broadside. She was killed instantly.

One wonders when another Helen Taussig will grace our planet. Her nimble brain and tireless dedication saved lives and prevented countless tragedies. She shared tears with the parents of her patients, and she shared the joy of discovery with her medical comrades. Best of all, she simply cared.

On a separate sheet of paper list all the underlined words in the story about Helen Taussig. Find them in the vocabulary section beginning on page 67. Review their meaning and pronunciation. Choose any four and write a sentence for each one.

HELEN BROOKE TAUSSIG
Vocabulary

LESSON NO. 1

Many small words can be made from large words. Follow the directions to make small words using the letters in the word "stethoscope." You do NOT have to use the letters in the order in which they appear in the word.

S T E T H O S C O P E

Find 2 words that end in "ope."

_____   _____

Find 2 five-letter words.

_____   _____

Find 2 words that end in "ot."

_____   _____

Find 2 words that begin with "sh."

_____   _____

Now try this word.

S P E C I A L I S T

Find 2 words that end in "ape."

_____   _____

Find 2 five-letter words.

_____   _____

Find 1 six letter word.

_____   _____

Find 2 words that begin with "cl."

_____   _____

Find 2 words that end with "ice."

_____   _____

HELEN BROOKE TAUSSIG
Activities

LESSON NO. 2

In Class

1. Write a letter to your local American Heart Association asking for: (1) a speaker to come to talk to the class about the causes and prevention of heart failure and (2) any written information they can send on the topic of heart problems.

2. Dr. Taussig believed that a good low-fat diet should begin in early childhood. Make a list of everything you ate yesterday and compare notes. Just how healthy is your diet?

At Home

1. List at least 5 common expressions that use the word "heart" (example: heart-to heart talk; heartbroken; heartthrob).

   _____

   _____

   _____

   _____

   _____

2. See if you can take the pulse of a family member (thumb laid lightly on inside of the wrist). Have someone take yours. Try to determine how many times one's heart beats in a minute.

At the Library

1. Today we hear a lot about heart bypass operations. See if you can locate material with diagrams that explains just what is involved in a heart bypass operation.

2. Find out what the prefix "dys" means, as in "dyslexia."

JONAS SALK
Children's Benefactor

The Problem

In the first half of this century parents were terrified that their children might get the <u>virus</u> called polio. It seemed to strike mostly in the summer months. Some years were worse than others. Many children grew sick and died. It was felt that the virus was more likely to attack in the hot, crowded cities. So those who could afford it fled to the country. Some cities were almost empty in the summer.

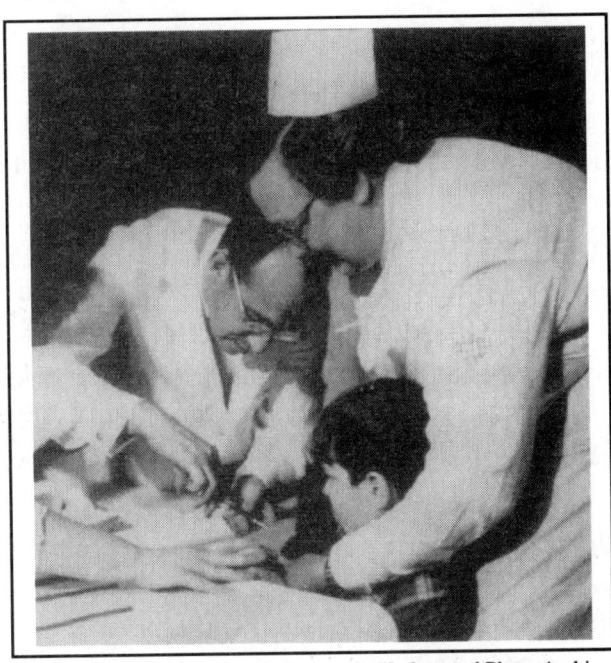

. . . Underwood Photo Archives

If one were unlucky enough to get this virus and live, the results were awful indeed. Some people (mostly children) became <u>paralyzed</u>. They could not move arms or legs or both. They would spend the rest of their lives on crutches or in wheelchairs. Others could not breathe without help. This meant they had to be moved into an "iron lung." This was a machine that forced air in and out of their lungs. They would have to face spending their lives in the iron lung. There was little hope for the future. No wonder the large cities were filled with panic during the long, hot summers.

The Solution

For years scientists had been working hard to find a way to prevent polio. Their task was not an easy one. By this time they knew how the body fought disease. And they knew quite a bit about polio. What they did not know was how to make a <u>vaccine</u> to fight the dread disease.

One of the many men working in labs on this problem was Jonas Salk. He and others knew that live polio virus had to be killed to make a vaccine. This was necessary so that the vaccine itself would not make people sick. Yet the virus had to remain active enough to produce <u>antibodies</u> that would fight off this disease. Who was Jonas Salk? How did he happen to be in the forefront of polio research?

Salk was born in New York City in 1914, the eldest of three sons. His father worked in the clothing trade. The family was not poor. But they certainly were not rich. Salk had to take after-school jobs to help pay for his education. He also earned a number of <u>scholarships</u>.

He first went to the City College of New York. Then he went on to the New York University School of Medicine. He <u>interned</u> for two years at Mount Sinai Hospital. By then he knew that he did not want to be a doctor who saw patients. He wanted to go into research. Things that went on in a lab fascinated him. One of his teachers got him a job in the University of Michigan lab at Ann Arbor. There he began to work on a flu vaccine. In those days flu often raged in <u>epidemics</u> and killed many people.

After five years had passed, Salk wanted a lab of his own. By this time he had a wife and three sons. Income was important. He moved his family to Pittsburgh. At once he became involved in a study of three strains of polio. The money for this work came from the National Foundation for Infantile Paralysis (another name for polio). This foundation was very well known. And there was a reason for this. The President of the United States had had polio. He could not walk without aid although he did his best to cover up that fact. He gave the National Foundation for Infantile Paralysis his full support. Money began to pour in for research. The March of Dimes was begun to honor the President. Everyone was asked to send a dime to him at the White House. This was a perfect way to raise money for research. The National Foundation gave Salk and his team $1,700,000 for their polio project.

The work went on. One failure seemed to follow another. Salk would not give up. And then one day at last he came up with a killed virus vaccine. He felt so sure that it was safe and effective, he used it on his wife, his sons, some friends, and himself. Next came a mass test of the vaccine. It was used on 650,000 school children in 44 states. Each child received three <u>injections</u> of the vaccine. The results of the test were announced on April 12, 1955. The vaccine was safe! The vaccine worked! It was a triumph.

The joy did not last long. Two weeks later a child who had been given the vaccine fell ill with polio. Then another – and another – a total of 204. All of the vaccine used on the children who grew ill came from one company. The tests were stopped. They were started again when vaccine from all the other companies was tested. It was found to be safe. From that time on, all vaccine was tested by the government. Once the scare was over, parents rushed to have their children <u>vaccinated</u>. The results were truly remarkable. For example, in 1952 there were 58,000 new cases of polio. In 1962 there were just over 900. Today there are even fewer.

Salk received lots of honors. There was a <u>citation</u> from the President. He also was offered $10,000 from an insurance company. But he would not take any cash awards for himself. The honors were not important. The work was important. And he wanted to get back to it. He <u>founded</u> the Salk <u>Institute</u> for <u>Biological</u> Studies. People from all over the world travel there to study and do research.

Salk would be the first to tell you that his great breakthrough would not have happened without the fine work of many men before him. For example, no effective vaccine could be made until the polio virus could be grown in large quantities. This step was accomplished by Enders, Weller, and Robbins. In fact, this <u>achievement</u> brought them the Nobel Prize in 1954. Other men had found that there were three types of polio virus. It was then clear that a polio vaccine had to work against all three types. And two men at Yale added to the known facts. They proved that the polio virus circulated through the blood before it attacked the nervous system. This meant that timing was important. A vaccine had to be given early. Otherwise serious damage would result

One other man must be mentioned: Albert Sabin. Sabin developed a live virus vaccine against polio. This happened almost at the same time as Salk's killed virus vaccine. His vaccine turned out to be cheaper than Salk's. It was also easier to give. The Sabin vaccine was given by mouth instead of by injection. He was never to receive the fame of Jonas Salk. But it should be known that it is the Sabin vaccine that is given to most children today. Both men deserve our thanks and gratitude.

On a separate sheet of paper list all the underlined words in the story about Jonas Salk. Find them in the vocabulary section beginning on page 67. Review their meaning and pronunciation. Choose any four and write a sentence for each one.

JONAS SALK
Fact or Opinion

LESSON NO. 1

A fact is very different from an opinion but sometimes we confuse the two. A fact is something that really happened, that is true, that can be proved.

    Example: There are 50 states in the United States of America.

An opinion is a belief or feeling that is not necessarily based on truth or proof.

    Example: Spring is the best time of the year.

Some of the statements below are facts and some are opinions. Write an F in front of the facts. Write an O in front of the opinions. You may refer back to the story about Jonas Salk if you wish.

1. _____ An "iron lung" forces air in and out of the lungs.

2. _____ Big cities are dangerous in the summer months.

3. _____ Jonas Salk tried his polio vaccine on himself and his family.

4. _____ Albert Sabin developed a vaccine at almost the same time as Jonas Salk.

5. _____ If you are poor in childhood, you will probably become famous when you become an adult.

6. _____ Animals should not be used in research.

7. _____ President Franklin Delano Roosevelt had polio.

8. _____ Drug companies are more interested in making a profit than in helping people.

9. _____ The work of many scientists helped Jonas Salk and Albert Sabin.

10. _____ Infantile paralysis is another name for polio.

11. _____ Most scientists get rich.

12. _____ Polio has been almost completely stamped out thanks to Jonas Salk and Albert Sabin.

JONAS SALK
Activities

LESSON NO. 2

In Class

1. Write a letter to the National Easter Seals Society, 230 W. Monroe Street, Chicago, Illinois 60606 and ask them if they have any printed information on polio they might send you.

2. Discuss what has been done in the community to make life easier for people in wheelchairs (ramps, wider doorways, etc.). What still needs to be done?

At Home

1. Check with parents to learn whether you were given the Salk or the Sabin vaccine. Bring the results to class. Tabulate to see how many received the Salk vaccine, how many the Sabin vaccine.

2. Write a short note to Jonas Salk thanking him for his great work on the polio vaccine and telling what it means to you.

At the Library

1. Study the life of President Franklin Delano Roosevelt. How old was he when he contracted polio? What disabling effects did it leave? How did he deal with them?

2. See if you can find out what research is currently underway at the Salk Institute for Biological Studies. You may have to seek out the address and write them.

CHRISTIAAN BARNARD
Maker of Medical History

The Problem

Before 1967 every doctor who dealt with heart patients knew that now and then he or she would encounter a case for which there was no cure, no hope. These were hearts that were simply worn out. Or perhaps they had been destroyed by <u>coronary</u> disease. After all, the heart is just a pump. When its pumping ability fails, the heart is useless. Life ceases.

Through the years major heart surgery improved. For example, surgeons were able to replace diseased heart valves with <u>artificial</u> valves. But many times they had to lose a patient when all that was really needed was a new pump. In other words, a new heart!

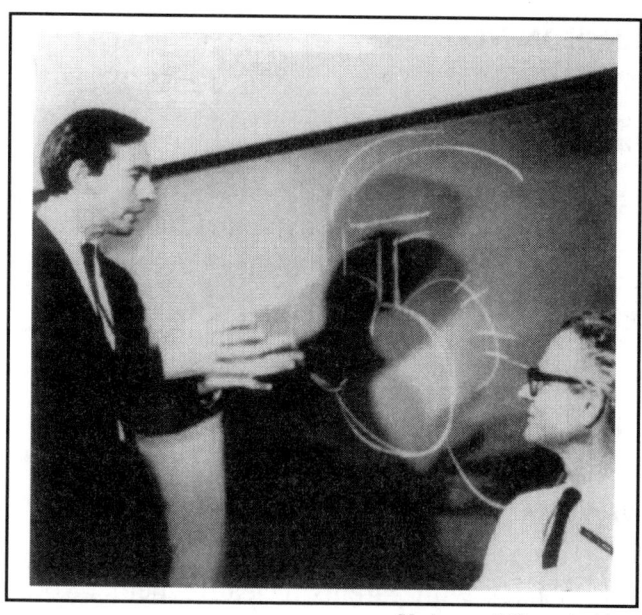

... Underwood Photo Archives

The Solution

The idea of replacing a worn-out heart with a new one had been considered for many years. But it was a daring surgeon in South Africa who decided that the time had come to try to transplant a heart. His name was Christiaan Barnard. Dr. Barnard had first to find a patient whose heart was badly diseased. It had to be someone for whom there was no hope. It didn't take long to find such a man. Louis Washansky was a 54-year-old grocer. He was dying of heart disease. He also had <u>diabetes</u> and an infection in one leg. He and his family agreed to a heart transplant. They really had no other choice.

The next step was to find a heart <u>donor</u>. Dr. Barnard and his 30-man team went on 24-hour alert. Whenever a heart was found, they had to be ready to spring into action. The first possible donor was a boy who had died in a car accident. After study this heart was rejected because it had been damaged by the effects of the accident. Then a young woman was killed crossing the street. Her blood type and Washansky's matched. The transplant team moved fast. There had to be two operations. One team was to remove the donor's heart. Another team was to prepare Washansky for a new heart. Everything had to be timed to a split second. The entire <u>procedure</u> went very well. Electric shock was used to get the new heart beating. Washansky had survived the incredible operation.

There was yet another problem. A new heart is a foreign organism in a body. The body's white cells try to reject it. To stop the rejection Washansky was given massive doses of drugs. This did stop the rejection. But it did something else. The drugs left Washansky's body helpless against infection. He became ill with double <u>pneumonia</u>. The transplant team stood sadly by. There was nothing they could do. Washansky died 18 days after the operation.

Who was Christiaan Barnard who dared to try something so likely to fail? He was born in a small village, the son of a poorly-paid minister. He had three brothers. The family was desperately poor. Dr. Barnard recalls that his Christmas stocking never held anything but a few pieces of candy. He also recalls that all of his clothes were hand-me-downs until he went to college. Until that time he didn't even know what size he wore!

Dr. Barnard was given a <u>scholarship</u> to the Medical School at the <u>University</u> of Cape Town in South Africa. But he was warned. Low grades in any course would cause him to lose the scholarship. After graduation he opened a practice in a small town. But research called. He was thrilled to get a research <u>fellowship</u> in surgery at Cape Town University. It was not an easy life. During the day he saw patients. At night from 10:00 P.M. to 2:00 A.M. he did his research. The research <u>facilities</u> were poor. To get the animals he needed for research he had to drive to the local <u>pound</u>. By the time he got back to the lab with the dogs, he and his car were full of fleas!

After a while he grew tired of the lack of good equipment and enough space. He went to the United States where he found a new post. The labs at the Medical School at the University of Minnesota were excellent. The pay was small, hardly enough to live on. Dr. Barnard mowed lawns, washed cars, and did other odd jobs. Before long though he received a sizable grant. Now he was able to finish his studies. He received an advanced degree in two years. During his stay in Minnesota, he did some <u>pioneer</u> work in birth defects. But heart research was his first love. So he returned to Cape Town as director of surgical research there. And more and more he grew interested in the possibility of heart transplants.

After the first heart transplant one of the American TV networks flew Dr. Barnard to the United States. He appeared on a number of important television shows and visited President Johnson at his Texas ranch. He returned home by way of Europe. Everywhere he went he was honored and treated as a <u>celebrity</u>.

It was time to look for another transplant patient. This time Dr. Barnard chose Philip Blaiberg, a 58-year-old retired dentist. The donor was a 24-year-old stroke victim. The second transplant operation went more smoothly than the first. Dr. Barnard had learned a lot about drugs from the Louis Washansky case. Dr. Blaiberg was given much smaller quantities of drugs. He was kept in the hospital for 74 days in a germ-free room. When he left the hospital, he was "smiling and happy." This was a great change from the dying man who had entered the hospital more than two months earlier. Later he became ill with hepatitis and a lung problem. But he lived until August 17, 1969, almost 20 months after the transplant.

That was the beginning of a whole new field of medicine. Today transplants are almost routine. Hearts and kidneys and other organs are regularly transplanted. Doctors seem to have found an answer to the problem of the body's rejecting a new organ. But today there is another problem. The supply of organs available for transplant is not equal to the demand. All too often people die while waiting for the needed organ to be located. To allow one's heart or kidney or other organ to be used after death to save another's life seems a very noble thing to do.

On a separate sheet of paper list all the underlined words in the story about Christiaan Barnard. Find them in the vocabulary section beginning on page 67. Review their meaning and pronunciation. Choose any four and write a sentence for each one.

CHRISTIAAN BARNARD
Syllables

LESSON NO. 1

All of these words have been taken from the story of Christiaan Barnard. Pronounce each word slowly. On the line in front of each word, write the number of syllables you heard. Remember: Each syllable must have one vowel sound.

_____ heart	_____ scholarship	_____ victim
_____ coronary	_____ graduation	_____ stroke
_____ disease	_____ grades	_____ routine
_____ surgery	_____ research	_____ available
_____ pump	_____ equipment	_____ encounter
_____ patient	_____ grant	_____ artificial
_____ diabetes	_____ pioneer	_____ woman
_____ transplant	_____ hospital	_____ blood
_____ accident	_____ hepatitis	_____ second
_____ donor	_____ kidneys	_____ organism
_____ operation	_____ doctor	_____ reject
_____ electric	_____ surgeon	_____ minister
_____ infection	_____ celebrity	_____ practice
_____ village	_____ animals	_____ university
_____ college	_____ medical	_____ pound

How many words did you find with 1 syllable? _____

with 2 syllables? _____

with 3 syllables? _____

with 4 syllables? _____

with 5 syllables? _____

Christiaan Barnard
Activities

LESSON NO. 2

In Class

1. Write a paragraph about which you would rather be: a surgeon, a plumber or a salesman. Give at least 5 reasons to support your choice.

2. Not too long ago Dr. Barnard's country abolished apartheid. (Apartheid: very strict racial segregation in schools, restaurants, theaters, churches, beaches, etc.) Divide into 2 teams and debate why versus why not this was a good thing for a country to do.

At Home

1. Pretend you are a TV commentator. You are going to announce the story of the first heart transplant on tonight's evening news. Write a script.

2. List the qualities a person must have to try something as unexplored and hazardous as the first organ transplant.

At the Library

1. Find out how many organs the body has and which of these can be transplanted.

2. Find out what steps must be taken if one wishes to make their heart or other organs available for transplant in case of sudden death.

VOCABULARY

VOCABULARY

achievement
(ə chēv′ mənt)

a thing done successfully
Writing a book was his greatest achievement.

amputate
(ăm′ pyσο tāt)

to cut off, especially by surgery
After the accident, they had to amputate one of his legs.

anatomy
(ə năt′ ə mē)

study of the structure of an animal or plant
He studied the anatomy of a leaf.

anesthesiology
(ăn ĕs thē zē ŏl′ ə jē)

the science of giving anesthetics (substance which has the
power to deprive of feeling or sensation)
She decided to specialize in anesthesiology.

antibody
(ăn′ tĭ bŏd ē)

any substance in the blood developed through immunization to
counteract toxins or bacterial poisons
A vaccination builds up smallpox antibodies.

antiseptic
(ăn tə sĕp′ tĭk)

agent that prevents growth of bacteria
She put some antiseptic on the cut.

appendicitis
(ə pĕn də sīt′ ĭs)

inflammation of a small sac attached to the large intestine
He was taken to the hospital with appendicitis.

application
(ăp lĭ kā shən)

a form asking for admission (job, school, etc.)
She filled out an application for the job.

apprentice
(ə prĕn′ tĭs)

a person being taught a craft or trade, now often a member of a
labor union
The blacksmith took him on as an apprentice.

approbation
(ăp rə bā′ shən)

approval; praise
The fans roared their approbation.

artificial
(ärt ə fĭsh′ əl)

not real or genuine
The stone in her ring was artificial.

67

astonish
(ə stŏn′ ĭsh)

to fill with sudden surprise or wonder
I was astonished by her performance.

bacteria
(băk tĭr′ ē ə)

micro-organisms that can cause disease or fermentation
There was bacteria growing on the stale bread.

bacteriologist
(băk tĭr′ ē ŏl′ ə jĭst)

one who works with micro-organisms that can cause disease or fermentation
She was a bacteriologist.

barricade
(bər′ ə kād)

a fence or barrier quickly built to stop an enemy
The soldiers raised a barricade to keep out the enemy.

biological
(bī ō lŏj′ ə kəl)

having to do with origin, habits, and characteristics of plants and animals
He majored in biological studies.

boundless
(bound′ lĭs)

unlimited; vast; great numbers or quantities
There seemed to be boundless quantities of food.

bypass
(bī′ păs)

a very delicate heart operation
He needed a heart bypass operation.

carbolic acid
(kär băl′ ĭk ă′ sĭd)

a chemical used to kill bacteria, etc.
Perhaps carbolic acid will kill the germs.

cardiology
(kär dē äl′ ə jē)

branch of medicine dealing with the heart
She specializes in cardiology.

celebrity
(sə lĕb′ rə tē)

a famous person
Queen Elizabeth is a celebrity.

cholera
(käl′ ər ə)

a serious infectious disease
Before his trip he was given a shot for cholera.

cholesterol
(kə lĕs′ tär ŏl)

a crystalline form of alcohol present in body cells and animal fats and tissues
My cholesterol is too high.

citation
(sī tā′ shən)

an official notice or honor
The governor gave him a citation for service to the state.

civilized
(sĭv′ ə līzd)

to come out of primitive conditions to a higher standard of living
The United States of America is a civilized country.

college
(käl′ ĭ j)

an institution of higher education
After high school, he went to college.

commission
(kə mĭsh′ ən)

a group formed to perform certain duties or tasks
The president appointed a commission to study children's health.

compensation
(käm pĕn sā′ shən)

payment
The compensation was too small for that difficult job.

complicated
(käm′ plĭ kā tĭd

hard to solve; difficult to comprehend
These directions are too complicated.

coronary
(kör′ ə nĕr ē)

pertaining to either or both of the two arteries of the heart
He was in the hospital after his coronary attack.

Crimea
(Krī mē ə)

a peninsula between the Black Sea and the Sea of Azov
The Crimea is a difficult place to get to.

curiosity
(kyoor ē äs′ ə tē)

desire to learn or discover something new
Curiosity killed the cat!

decision
(dē sĭzh′ shən)

final judgment or opinion; firm statement or conclusion
Please make a decision today.

dedication
(dĕd ĭ kā′ shən)

devotion to a special project or specific purpose (also dedicated)
Her dedication to her job is admirable.

delegate
(dĕl′ ə gət)

a person sent to represent others at a special meeting or convention
He was a delegate to the national conference.

device
(dĭ vīs′)

something invented for a special use
An electric can-opener is a helpful device.

diabetes
(dī ə bĕt′ ēz)

a chronic disease characterized by excessive sugar in the blood and urine
She suffers from diabetes.

dissect
(dī sĕkt′)

to cut apart piece by piece
The assignment was to dissect a frog.

distinguished
(dĭ stĭn′ gwĭsht)

separated from others by extraordinary qualities; famous
The president of our company is a distinguished woman.

donated
(dō′ nāt ĕd)

given; contributed
He donated $500 to the building fund.

donor
(dō′ nər)

one who gives or makes a contribution
He was a regular blood donor.

dyslexic
(dĭs lĕk′ sĭk)

one who has difficulty learning to read
The teacher decided he was dyslexic.

encourage
(ĕn kër′ ĭj)

to give support to; to stimulate or help
She encouraged him to get a tutor.

engineer
(ĕn jə nĭr′)

one skilled in some branch of technology
The engineer was working on the blueprints.

epidemic
(ĕp ə dĕm′ ĭk)

spreading rapidly among many people in a community, as a disease
The town had an epidemic of flu.

ether
(ē′ thər)

a highly flammable colorless liquid used as an anesthetic
They gave my son ether when they removed his tonsils.

extract
(ĕks trăkt′)

to draw out or pull out by effort
The dentist extracted a wisdom tooth.

facility
(fə sĭl′ ə tē)

a building or room used for a particular purpose, such as a laboratory
The factory needed a new heating facility.

faculty
(făk′ əl tē)

all of the teachers at a school or one of its departments
Our school has an outstanding faculty.

fellowship
(fĕl′ ō shĭp)

money given for the support of a student doing advanced work
He was given a fellowship to Oxford.

ferment
(fur měnt′)

to cause a substance to undergo a change
We are waiting for the wine to ferment.

foreigner
(för′ ĭn ər)

a person from another country
Foreigners bring a lot of new ideas to our country.

found
(found)

to set up; establish; start
He founded a new hospital.

genius
(jēn′ yəs)

great mental and creative ability
Einstein was a genius.

graduate
(gră′ jo͞o āt)

to complete a course of study at a school or college
I graduated from high school.

hurdle
(hurd′ l)

an obstacle to be overcome
The runner leaped over the hurdle.

hygiene
(hī′ jēn)

cleanliness; system to preserve health
Good hygiene is always important for good health.

immortal
(ĭm mört′ l)

living forever
The music of Mozart is immortal.

immune
(ĭm myo͞on′)

free or protected from something harmful such as a disease
After my shots I am now immune to polio.

imperturbable
(ĭm pər tur′ bə bəl)

calm; collected
Her manner is always imperturbable.

industrial
(ĭn dŭs′ trē əl)

having to do with manufacturing or factories
He lived in a large industrial section of town.

inequality
(ĭn ē kwol′ ĭ tē)

the condition of being unequal
Inequality of race must be eliminated.

infirmary
(ĭn fur′ mə rē)

a place for the care of the sick
She was taken to an infirmary to recover.

injection
(ĭn jěkt′ shən)

act of introducing a liquid into the body with a syringe; a shot
It is time for your iron injection.

institute
(ĭn′ stə tōōt)

a school, often within a university, specializing in highly technical studies
I am enrolled in the institute for foreign languages.

intern
(ĭn′ turn)

a doctor working as assistant in a hospital generally just after graduation from medical school
He will spend 3 years at the hospital as an intern.

knighted
(nīt′ əd)

in England to be given an honorary rank with the privilege of using "Sir" before a given name. Example: Sir Walter Raleigh
He was thrilled when he heard he was to be knighted by the Queen.

lecture
(lĕk′ chər)

an informative talk to a class or audience
I can't be late for my chemistry lecture.

legendary
(lĕj′ ən dĕr ē)

famous or described in fictional stories or historical fact
Galahad is a legendary figure.

liberal
(lĭb′ ər əl)

one who favors progress; tolerant; broad-minded
I am proud to be a liberal.

lowly
(lō′ lē)

humble; meek; low position in life
He held a very lowly job.

mentally retarded
(mĕn′ təl lē   rĭ tärd əd)

a handicapping condition indicated by slower than normal learning, development, and social adjustment.
The class was formed for mentally retarded children.

mucus
(myōō′ kəs)

a thick fluid secreted by membranes of the body
A cold generally causes a great deal of mucus.

mysterious
(mĭs tĭr′ ē əs)

not explained or revealed; beyond human comprehension
Her disappearance is very mysterious.

native
(nāt′ ĭv)

belonging to a country by birth; an original inhabitant
He is a native of Pakistan.

normal
(nôr′ məl)

conforming to an accepted standard; natural; usual
His growth seems to be normal for his age.

nuclear
(noo̅′ klē ər)

pertaining to the use of atomic energy
All countries are trying to avoid a nuclear war.

obstacle
(ŏb′ stə kəl)

anything that stands in the way
The poor child had many obstacles to overcome.

occupation
(ŏk yoo̅ pā′ shən)

one's work or profession
I am thinking of changing my occupation.

ophthamology
(ŏf thăl mŏl′ ō jē)

the medical science that deals with diseases of the eye
My eye doctor studied ophthamology for many years.

oxygen
(ŏks′ ĭ jən)

a colorless, odorless, gaseous chemical element; essential to life
Water consists of oxygen and hydrogen.

paralysis
(pə răl′ ə sĭs)

loss of the power to move one or more parts of the body
After the accident he suffered from paralysis of his legs.

pasteurization
(păs chě rīz ā′ shən)

the process of destroying bacteria by heating to a prescribed temperature for a specified time
Pasteurization of milk has saved many lives.

pathology
(pə thŏl′ ə jē)

the science that deals with the nature and causes of disease
The doctors discussed the pathology of the case.

peculiar
(pē kyoo̅l′ yər⁻)

odd; strange
That is a peculiar odor in the lab.

pediatric
(pē dē ă′ trĭk)

the branch of medicine that deals with the care and treatment of infants and children
She wants to become a pediatric nurse.

penicillin
(pĕn ĭ sĭl′ ĭn)

an antibiotic produced from certain molds
Sir Alexander Fleming discovered penicillin.

perfecting
(pur fĕkt′ ĭng)

completing; finishing; improving; bringing to completion
He is busy perfecting his new process.

pioneer
(pī ə nĭr′)

one who goes before and prepares the way for others
The pioneers settled in the West.

plight
(plīt)

a distressing situation
When the boat sank, the passengers were in a terrible plight.

pneumonia
(noo mōn′ yə)

disease; inflammation of the lungs caused by bacteria or viruses
First I had a cold, then pneumonia.

post-graduate
(pōst - grǎ′ joo ĭt)

one who engages in advanced studies after graduation from college
Next year I begin my post-graduate work at the university.

post-operative
(pōst - ŏp′ ər ə tĭv)

occurring after a surgical operation
Her post-operative care is very important.

post-surgical
(pōst - sur′ jĭ kəl)

same as post-operative above
Her post-surgical care is very important.

pound
(pound)

a place where stray animals are kept
We found our great dog at the pound.

principles
(prĭn′ sə pəlz)

a method or rule of conduct; integrity
She is a person of high principles.

procedure
(prō sē′ jər)

a particular course of action
Please tell me what procedure to follow.

proposal
(prō pōz′ əl)

a plan or suggestion
His proposal made a lot of sense.

pus
(pŭs)

a yellow-white thick substance found in infected sores and wounds
Did the wound have any pus in it?

rabid
(rǎb′ ĭd)

having rabies
Everyone ran from the rabid dog.

rabies
(rā′ bēz)

a disease people get from the bite of an infected animal; can be fatal unless treatment is started early.
The series of rabies shots was very painful.

radical
(rǎd′ ĭ kəl)

favoring basic change, sometimes extreme
His views are somewhat radical.

radiology
(rā dē ŏl′ ə jē)

the use of x-rays in medical diagnosis and therapy
I was sent to the department of radiology.

reason
(rē′ zən)

to think out logically
It is best to reason things out slowly and carefully.

regularity
(rĕg yə lĕr′ ĭ tē)

orderly; consistent; conforming to what is usual or normal
He seems to be late with great regularity.

repulsive
(rĭ pŭls′ ĭv)

disgusting; causing strong dislike
The Halloween mask was repulsive.

responsible
(rĭ spŏn′ sə bəl)

meeting one's obligations or duties; reliable; dependable
She is extremely responsible.

rheumatic fever
(rōōm ă′ tĭk fē′ vər)

a serious disease, usually of children, with fever, swelling of the joints, inflammation of the heart, etc.
He recovered from rheumatic fever.

scholarship
(skäl′ ər shĭp)

a gift of money to help a student pay college expenses
She was thrilled when she got a college scholarship.

scholastic
(skə lăs′ tĭk)

pertains to schools or education
Her scholastic achievement is outstanding.

shambles
(shăm′ bəlz)

a place or scene of great disorder; a mess
The house was in shambles.

site
(sīt)

location; the scene of an event
They chose a site for their new home.

specialist
(spĕsh′ əl ĭst)

one who knows a great deal about one particular subject; in medicine one who devotes himself to a particular class of diseases
She is a specialist in children's diseases.

specimen
(spĕs′ ə mən)

a sample; an organism preserved as an example of its kind
That is a perfect specimen of a fossil.

staph
(stăf)

short for staphylococcus, a form of bacteria which causes illness
He got a staph infection from eating bad hamburger.

stethoscope
(stĕth′ ə skōp)

an instrument used to examine heart, lungs, etc., by listening to the sounds they make
The doctor put on her stethoscope and listened to his heart.

strep throat
(strĕp thrōt)

short for streptococcus, a bacteria which can cause a serious disease
He missed a lot of school because he had strep throat.

strike
(strīk)

to refuse to continue work until certain demands are met.
The workers went out on strike.

superintendent
(soo pər ĭn tĕn′ dənt)

a person in charge of a department or institution
He held the position of superintendent of schools.

superstition
(soo pər stĭsh′ ən)

any belief that is not consistent with known facts; belief in omens
Believing that Friday the 13th is unlucky is a superstition.

system
(sĭs′ təm)

a set of facts arranged to show a plan; an orderly way of doing something
I have a new system of studying for a test.

technical
(tĕk′ nĭ kəl)

a specific science, craft, art, etc.; concerned with tiny details
The engineer had a lot of technical information.

technique
(tĕk nēk′)

method of proceeding in scientific activity, artistic work, etc.
I admired the ballet dancer's technique.

texture
(tĕks′ chər)

the surface structure of an object
The cloth had a rough texture.

theory
(thē′ ə rē)

an arrangement of facts; principles of science
The detective had a theory about the crime.

tissue
(tĭsh′ oo)

substance of an organic body, consisting of cells, etc.
We needed a tissue sample for the test.

toxic
(tŏks′ ĭk)

poisonous
Everyone fears a toxic spill.

tragic
(trăj′ ĭk)

disastrous; extremely sad
She came to a tragic end.

translate
(trăns lāt′)

to put into the words of a different language
Please translate this from English to French.

tropical
(trŏp′ ĭ kəl′)

very hot (sometimes diseases related to the tropics)
I like living in a tropical climate.

tsar
(zär)

(same as Czar) early ruler of Russia
Russia no longer has a tsar.

typical
(tĭp′ ĭ kəl)

conforming to some type; characteristic
He is a typical military man.

unanimous
(yo͞o năn′ ə məs)

agreeing completely in opinion; being of one mind
The vote was unanimous.

universal
(yo͞on ə vur′ səl)

used by all people
Hating war and seeking peace is a universal attitude.

university
(yo͞on ə vur′ sə tē)

an educational institution which offers advanced degrees
After high school she went to a university.

vaccinate
(văk′ sə nāt)

to inoculate with a vaccine to prevent disease
The doctor will vaccinate you for smallpox.

vaccine
(văk sēn′)

a substance used to produce immunity to a specific disease
They ran out of smallpox vaccine.

veterinary
(vĕt′ ər ə nĕr ē)

the branch of medicine that deals with animals
She is studying veterinary medicine.

virtually
(vur′ cho͞o əl lē)

almost entirely
That road is virtually finished.

virus
(vĭ′ rəs)

any of a large group of infective agents that cause disease
Many people have come down with the flu virus.

vow
(vou)

a solemn promise
They made a vow to be friends always.

will
(wĭl)

determination; strong desire
He will succeed because he has a will to get ahead.